B.H.M.S.
STUDENT'S GUIDE
TO
PRACTICE OF MEDICINE

B.H.M.S.
STUDENT'S GUIDE
TO
PRACTICE OF MEDICINE

DR. RITU ARORA
B.H.M.S.
N.H.M.C., NEW DELHI

B. Jain Publishers (P) Ltd.
An ISO 9001 : 2000 Certified Company
USA—EUROPE—INDIA

STUDENT'S GUIDE TO PRACTICE OF MEDICINE

First Edition: 1992
7th Impression: 2009

NOTE FROM THE PUBLISHERS
Any information given in this book is not intended to be taken as a replacement for medical advice. Any person with a condition requiring medical attention should consult a qualified practitioner or therapist.

All rights reserved. No part of this book may be reproduced, stored in a retrieval system or transmitted, in any form or by any means, mechanical, photocopying, recording or otherwise, without any prior written permission of the publisher.

© with the publisher

Published by Kuldeep Jain for
B. JAIN PUBLISHERS (P) LTD.
An ISO 9001 : 2000 Certified Company
1921/10, Chuna Mandi, Paharganj, New Delhi 110 055 (INDIA)
Tel.: 91-11-2358 0800, 2358 1100, 2358 1300, 2358 3100
Fax: 91-11-2358 0471 • *Email:* info@bjain.com
Website: **www.bjainbooks.com**

Printed in India by
Akash Press
ISBN: 978-81-319-0774-0

FOREWORD

I had the privilege of knowing Dr. Ritu Arora very closely for a number of years. Members of teaching faculty always admired her lucidity of thoughts and comprehensive knowledge of the subject discussed in theoretical and clinical classes. She has meticulously answered almost all the important questions.

Her main achievement in this book has been to corelate the theoretical concepts and practical needs of the students. For more curious students, some rare, lesser known drugs have also been mentioned in addition to the common ones.

I am confident that the objective of the most important aspect of Practice of Medicine will be admirably achieved by this authoritative book.

I congratulate the author for her valuable work.

New Delhi
11-8-1992

Dr. V.K. KHANNA
Asstt. Professor
Nehru Homoeopathic
Medical College & Hospital
New Delhi-110 024

PREFACE

It gives me an immense pleasure to present this book to the students appearing for final B.H.M.S. Examination. It has been written in a most concised, compact, to the point and lucid manner. While writing this book, I have constantly kept in mind the requirements of all the students regarding the latest as well as the changing trends of their examination.

In short, it is expected that the book will prove to be an asset for the students.

Despite the best efforts put in by me, it is possible that some unintentional errors might have eluded me. I shall acknowledge with gratitude any such errors, if pointed out. Any suggestions from students and colleagues for improvement in future editions of this book are most welcome.

In the end, I shall not forget to thank Dr. P.N. Jain, Mg. Director, of M/s. B. Jain Publishers for giving me this opportunity.

New Delhi
11-8-1992

DR. RITU ARORA

Contents

Sl. No.	System Discussed	Page No.
	Foreword	iii
	Preface	iv
1.	Pediatrics	1
2.	Skin	11
3.	Liver and Gall Bladder	29
4.	Bones and Joints	47
5.	Excretory System	60
6.	Endocrine System	82
7.	Psychiatry	103
8.	Gastrointestinal System	111
9.	Nervous System	138
10.	Respiratory System	169
11.	Haemopoetic System	196
12.	Cardiovascular System	211
13.	Infectious, Tropical and Deficiency Diseases	233

1. PEDIATRICS

Q-1. Discuss the causes and symptoms of Cerebral Palsy Mention important drugs for its treatment. (1987, 1988)

Ans. Cerebral Palsy can be defined as a non progressive Neuro muscular disorder OF CEREBRAL ORIGIN.

CAUSES:
1. Cerebral Anoxia
2. Trauma to the Brain
3. Congenital malformations
4. Kern Icterus.
5. Infections ante or post natally
6. Metabolic Disorders: Hypoglycaemia

The Symptoms are usually very few but the manifestations depend on the site of lesion:

1. SPASTIC TYPE: About 65% of Children are spastic due to motor cortex involvement.
   Quadriplegia, hemiplegia or monoplegia with Hyper excitability, persistence of Neonatal reflexes, Scissoring gait, difficulty in swallowing and drooling of saliva.
2. EXTRAPYRAMIDAL TYPE: They include athetosis, Choreiform movements, tremors and LEAD PIPE RIGIDITY.
3. CEREBELLAR TYPE: Child comes with Ataxia - difficulty in walking and intention Tremors. On examination there is Hypotonia with Hypo Reflexia.

Besides these the following may be present:
1. EYES: The child may have strabismus, cataract or paralysis of gaze.

3. SPEECH: Aphasia, dysarthria and dyslalia are common presentations.
4. INTELLIGENCE: About a quarter of the children have borderline intelligence.

HOMOEOPATHIC MANAGEMENT:

1. BARYTA CARB: It is suited to those children who are scrofulous, mentally and physically backward, do not grow and develop, have swollen abdomen take cold easily always have swollen TONSILS.
   Suppurative tonsils from every cold, with swollen glands in the nape of neck.
2. HELLEBORUS: It is suited to the children of cerebellar involvement when there is general muscular weakness. There is involuntary sighing with constant picking of lips and bed clothes. There is rolling of head with chewing motion of the lower jaw.
   There is constant dribbling of saliva from the mouth.
3. ZINCUM METALLICUM: It is one of the excellent Remedies to be used in cerebral affections when BRAIN FAG is very well marked.
   The child suffers from convulsions with marked pallor and absence of heat during the attack.
   The causative factor usually in the background is suppressed eruptions, exanthema or suppressed discharges.
   The child suffers from empty all gone feeling in the stomach and is always better by eating.
   The child is very lethargic, stupid in appearance and repeats everything said to it.

Q-2. What is Hydrocephalus? Give its symptoms with the Homoeopathic management (1987).

Ans. DEFINITION: Hydrocephalus is a condition in which a portion of the entire ventricular system is abnormally dilated and the C.S.F is under the increased pressure.

It results from an imbalance between the production and absorption of C.S.F.

The symptoms can be studied under the following:

1. ENLARGED HEAD: The head is dispropotionately larger than the body. The head usually enlarges in proportion to the level of pressure of the fluid.

2. SEPARATED SUTURES : They get seperated and widened with fullness of Ant fontanelle.
3. PROMINENT SCALP VEINS: Due to increased drainage of the blood the superficial scalp veins become prominent.
4. SUN SETTING SIGN: There is downward displacement of the orbital plates which pushes the eyeballs down and a large portion of sclera is exposed. Along with it there is divergent squint.
5. RETARDED GROWTH: Both physical and the mental growth and development of the child is affected. Therefore he may be a physically handicapped and mentally retarded child.
6. NEUROLOGICAL MANIFESTATIONS: like spasticity of lower limbs, epileptic convulsions may be seen.

HOMOEOPATHIC MANAGEMENT

1. APIS MELLIFICA: It is speically suited to the scrofulous children who usually suffer from Dropsical effusion of the Brain. The child is very irritable and awkward and drop things from the hands.

    Whole brain feels tired child is thirstless but with craving for milk.

    Child constantly bores the head into pillow with CRY ENCEPHALIQUE. It is associated with a tendency for diarrhoea and dropsical effusions of serous cavities. The child is very drowsy but screams and starts during the sleep.

    Child is always better by cold bathing and in open air.

2. IODOFORMUM: It should be remembered when the cause is of Tubercular origin. There is usually a history of subacute attacks of diarrhoea in the childhood.

    The head is very large with sharp occipital pains but with scaphoid abdomen. Abdomen is distended with enlarged mesentric glands.

    Chronic diarrhoea with greenish watery stools with marked irritability. Child cannot stand and walk with eyes closed.

3. HELLEBORUS: It is suited to the children when there is a definite history of low vitality. The child sees, hears

tastes imperfectly with general muscular weakness. Child is thoughtless, staring with involuntary sighing, constant rubbing of nose with Automatic motion of one arm and leg. The child is always worse from 4-8 P.m.

4. ZINCUM METALLICUM : See Q-1

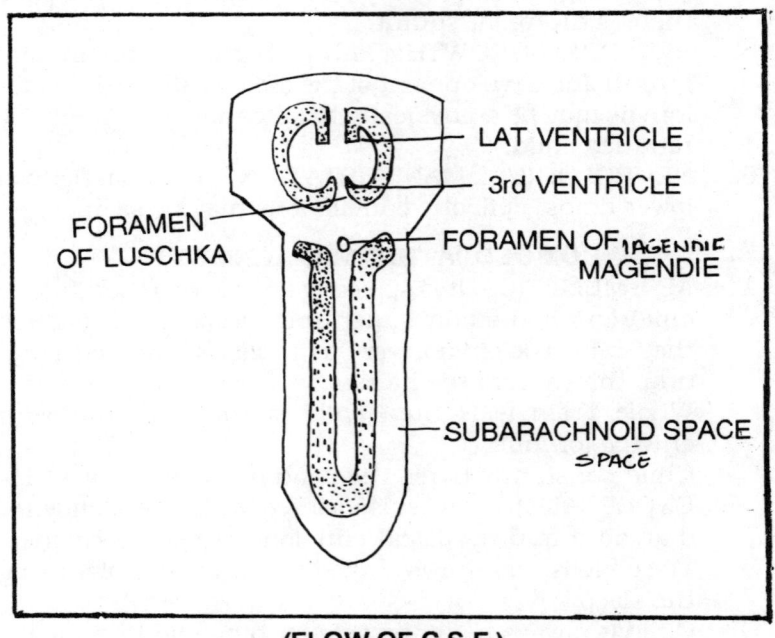

(FLOW OF C.S.F.)

Q-3. Discuss in details about diarrhoea in the infants. Give the differential diagnosis with general management (1982, 1983, 1985).

Ans. Diarrhoea is a common but potentially serious illness in the early childhood. On an average a child suffers from 10-15 episodes of diarrhoea in first five years of

ETIOLOGY:

Most of the cases are usually due to the action of micro-organisms specially bacteria which act in the 2 ways:
1. Through the toxins released.
2. By direct invasion of intestinal mucosa.

The organims responsible are:
A. BACTERIA: E. Coli, Campylobacter, Shigella etc.
B. VIRUSES: Rota Visuses, Adenovirus etc.
C. PARASITES: E. Histolytica, Giardia etc.

CLINICAL MANIFESTATIONS:

1. MILD CASE: Onset with loose diarrhoeal type of stools. Stools are usually greenish, slightly offensive with mucus; varying in number from 2-3 to 10-12 per day.
2. SEVERE CASE: Onset is moderately severe with or without vomiting. Stools are usually watery and odourless. Dehydration sets in early with evidence of in-

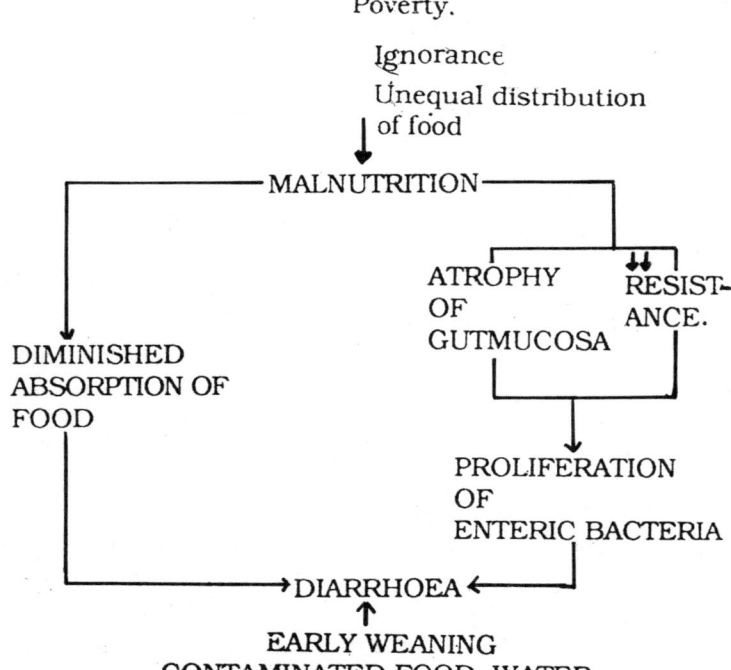

creased thirst, dry tongue, depressed fontanelle, tachycardia. oliguria and loss of elasticity of the skin.

Later symptoms of toxaemia like staring sunken eyes, apathy, shallow respiration, high temperature are seen.

GENERAL MANAGEMENT:

1. CORRECTION OF DEHYDRATION: The Correction is done according to the grades of dehydration.
   For this following can be used :
   a. Ringer Lactate: Full strength 1 : 20 with 5% glucose is used.
   b. Glucose Saline: It is given Intravenously.
2. DIET: Clear fluids containing electrolytes are given in the first 24 hours. After some hours weak milk mixture may be substituted.
   Besides this, boiled and mashed potato, mashed bananas, curd, butter milk, boiled rice can be given at regulated intervals in a regulated quantity.
3. REMOVAL OF TOXIC MATERIAL FROM THE BOWELS: Although in routine cases of mild severity it is not required But in cases of severity the bowel wash with a weak condy's solution can be given.
   It can be substituted by Stomach wash if vomiting is present especially with mucus.

HOMOEOPATHIC MANAGEMENT:

1. ALOES: It is a very good remedy for re establishing physiological equilibrium after much dosing. Abdomen feels full heavy, hot and bloated.
   The stools are loose with jelly like mucus with pain in rectum after stool.
   The stools are always associated with intense flatulence. Child constantly desires feed after stools.
2. PODOPHYLLUM: It is specially suited to the children of billious temprament.
   It is suitable for diarrhoea of long standing when the stools are profuse, polychromatic, putrid with prolapse of rectum and painless in nature.
   It is also useful in Dentition diarrhoea with hot, glowing cheeks and constant desire to press the gums together.

Child is always aggravated in the morning and in hot weather.
3. ARSENIC ALBUM: It is specially suited to those children who are extremely weak, punny and very restless. The Complaints are usually periodical in nature. The stools are usually offensive, dark with much prostration, scanty with blood.
Child is always aggravated by eating and drinking and after midnight specially 12-2 A.M.
There is burning thirst for water with icy coldness of the whole body.

DIFFERENTIAL DIAGNOSIS:
1. DEFICIENCY OF BILE SALTS:
a. Liver Diseases:- Choledochal cyst, hepatitis, infantile cirrhosis.
b. Bile duct Atresia.
c. Intestinal Stasis.
2. DEFICIENCY OF PANCREATIC ENZYMES:
a. Cystic Fibrosis.
b. Chronic pancreatitis.
3. MULTIPLE DEFECTS OF DIGESTION AND ABSORPTION:
a. Cow's milk allergy.
b. Enteritis
c. Coeliac Disease
4. DEFECTS OF CHYLOMICRONS:
a. Lymphoma
b. Lymphangectasis of intestines.

Q-4. Describe the functions of Thyroid gland. Discuss the clinical manifestations of Hypothyroid gland occuring in a child. How will you treat the case Homoeopathically? (1982 Supp.)

Ans. Thyroid is one of the important endocrine glands of the body. They are pair of glands with 2 lobes that are united by an Isthmus.

FUNCTIONS OF THYROID GLAND:
1. METABOLISM: It stimulates the metabolism of carbohydrates, fats and protein along with the metabolism of

Iodine and minerals like calcium and phosphorus.
2. GROWTH AND DIFFERENTIATION: The growth is influenced by the Growth Hormone of pitutiary.
It helps in the skeletal, muscular, sexual and the mental growth.
3. INFLUENCE ON CARDIOVASCULAR SYSTEM: It causes an increase in the systolic B.P without any alteration in the diastolic. It also increases the stroke volume. Cardiac irritability and output and causes the dilatation of peripheral vessels.
4. INFLUENCE ON NERVOUS SYSTEM: It increases the senstivity of the Nervous system.
5. MATURATION OF R.B.C: It indirectly influences the metabolism of vit B_{12} and Folic acid thereby, helps in the maturation of red cells.
6. HEAT REGULATION: The thyroxine has a CALORIGENIC effect thereby helps in the heat regulation.
7. SECRETION OF MILK: It stimulates and maintains the secretion of milk during lactation. It also increases the content of milk.

MANIFESTATIONS OF HYPOTHYROIDISM IN A CHILD:

It is called cretinism in children.

It usually results from relative or absolute deficiency of thyroxine.

The following are the features:
1. The Infant is dull and lethargic
2. Growth is retarded.
3. Large protruding tongue, broad flat nose, widely set eyes, sparse hairs, dry skin, protuberant abdomen and increased evidence of unbilical Hernia.
4. Abnormal persistence of physiological jaundice, croaky voice, constipation, somnolence and problems in feeding.
5. NEUROLOGICAL ABNORMALITIES:
a. Deafness b. Spastic limbs   c. At times coma.
6. Severely retarded mental development.
7. BONE CHANGES: The appearance and ossification of several epihyseal centres are delayed. Delayed eruption of teeth.

8. Associated Syndromes:
a. Hoffman's Syndrome: Hypertrophy of muscles associated with Pseodomyotonia.
b. Pendred's Syndrome: It is a congenital Syndrome when there is permanent deafness or deaf mutism with goitorous Hypothyrodism.
9. Neurological Signs:
a. Tendon Reflexes are altered
b. Relaxation phase is delayed.
c. Nerve conduction velocity is decreased.

HOMOEOPATHIC MANAGEMENT:

1. BARYTA MUR: The child is dwarf both physically and mentally. These children usually suffer from the defects of fat metabolism, therefore, with leading manifestations.

   Tonsils are generally enlarged with constant whizzing, buzzing in ears.

   It is associated with icy coldness of the body with paralysis and loss of voluntary muscle power.

   There is increased excretion of uric acid with diminished chlorides.

2. AETHUSA: The child is full of anguish, always crying with expression of uneasiness and discontent.

   There is well marked linea nasalis with a sunken expression of face.

   There is complete inability to digest milk with vomiting of milk and the same passes out in the stools.

   Child is unable to think, to fix attention any where with marked idiocy

   The body is usually covered with cold and clammy sweat.

3. IODUM: It is suited to the children of scrofulous variety who are dark complexioned, with enlarged lymphatic glands and usually of tubercular nature.

   There is sudden impulse to run and do violence but fear of people. He shuns everyone, sits in the corner doing nothing.

   The child is the HOTTEST patients in all with ravenous

hunger but losses flesh easily due to recurrent gastric and billiary upsets.

There are violent flushes of heat with intense sweating all over the body.

Q-5. Write short notes on:
a.   Crying baby and it's causes: (1990)
Ans. A baby born is really a creature who does not know how to express himself, to ask for help or to demand anything.

Therefore the only way God has gifted to him is the CRY. The cry of a baby always diverts the attention of the mother.

CAUSES:
1. HUNGER: When the baby is hungry he cries.
2. COLIC: When ever the baby has pain anywhere usually earache or belly ache he cries.
3. STARTLED FROM SLEEP: When the baby is suddenly startled or gets afraid, then weeps.
4. WET NAPPY: When the baby urinates or defecates, he calls the mother by crying.
5. ALONE: When the baby is alone and does not find anyone around him then makes itself known by its cry.

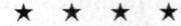

2. SKIN

Q-1. Discuss in detail Psoriasis with special mention of its articular complications. Mention the Homoeopathic treatment (1988).

Ans. *DEFINITION:* Psoriasis is a common chronic and non infectious skin disease characterised by well defined slightly raised, dry, erythematous macules with silvery scales.

ETIOLOGY:
No definite etiology is known.
  It is a Heredofamilial disease brought on by stress anxiety and mental trauma.
AGE: The commonest age is between 5-15 yrs.
WEATHER: It recurs in spring and autumn.
  It is seen more in dark haired persons.

PRECIPITATING FACTORS:
1. Child birth
2. Streptococcal Infections
3. Diabetes
4. Excessive purines in diet.

PATHOLOGY: It is a disorder of Keratinization. There are marked vascular changes in the upper dermis in the form of tortusity and dilatation.
  There is rapid replacement of epidermis.

CLINICAL FEATURES:
1. NATURE OF LESIONS: The lesions are well defined maculopapular type with layer of silvery scales over them.
   They are usually coin shaped; bilaterally symmetrical.
2. SITE: The typical distribution is on the Extensor sur-

face of the body, other areas like scalp, back of elbows, front of knee, legs and lower part of the back, nails, palms and soles are commonly affected.
3. ITCHING: Although there is no itching in majority but when associated with psychogenic stress and lichenification pruritus is very marked.
4. CANDLE GREASE SIGN: When the lesion is scratched with a forcep a candle grease like scale can be produced even from the non scaling lesions.
5. AUSPITZ SIGN: The complete removal of the scale produces pin point bleeding. It is called auspitz sign.

ARTICULAR COMPLICATIONS: In a long standing case of psoriasis, the joints like knee, or the small joints like those of hands are affected.

Psoriasis when affects the joints and complicates it is called PSORIATIC ARTHROPATHY.

It may manifest clinically as:
1. A symmetrical oligo arthritis.
2. Symmetrical Sero negative Arthritis.
3. Distal I.P. Joint arthritis.
4. Arthritis mutilans.
5. Sacroilitis or spondylitis.

DIAGNOSTIC FEATURES:

1. Lesions of psoriasis confined to areas like scalp, Natal cleft, umbilicus.
2. A family H/O psoriasis or joint involvement.
3. Nail changes: With subungal Hyperkeratosis
a. Pitting of Nails.
b. Seperation of distal portion of the nail from the nail bed.
c. Thickening of nails.
4. Involvement of distal I.P joints.
5. Moderately raised E.S.R.

HOMOEOPATHIC TREATMENT:

1. ARSENIC ALBUM: It is specially suited to those persons who are pale, emaciated, weak and irritable.

Skin is dry, scaly and rough with intense burning Psoriasis with itching which is usually worse from cold and at midnight.

Skin

Itching is worse by scratching.

2. **KALI ARS:** It is good when psoriasis has a tendency for chronicity, Intolerable itching which is worse when undressing. Psoriasis with intense lichenification.
Itching is worse from warmth, and from walking.
The patient is very restless and Nervous.

3. **PSORINUM:** It is suited to those persons who have latent psora which bursts out in the form of various skin affections particularly psoriasis.
Skin is dry, dirty with a dingy look.
There is intolerable itching which is worse from warmth of bed but better by covering.
The skin is very oily with excessive secretions of sebaceous glands. It perspires very easily on least exertion. All the complaints are worse in winters.

Q-2. Discuss Syphilis. Give its clinical features of all the 3 stages. Mention the Homoeopathic treatment. (1988 Supp).

Ans. *DEFINITION:* Syphilis is one of the commonest veneral diseases of infectious origin caused by a Treponema Pallidum.

It can affect any structure in the body and can mimic any disease.

ETIOLOGY:

It is caused by a spiral organism TREPONEMA PALLIDUM

MODE OF INFECTION: It can be

1. Direct: Usually by sexual intercourse kissing and fondling the genitalia can also affect it.
2. Indirect
3. Accidental
4. Congenital

CLINICAL FEATURES:

Clinically it can be studied under.
1. ACQUIRED   2. CONGENITAL.
ACQUIRED:
Early syphilis   Late Syphilis

a. Primary　　　　　　　　　a. Late Latent
b. Secondary　　　　　　　　b. Benign Tertiary
c. Early Latent　　　　　　　c. Cardiovascular Syphilis
　　　　　　　　　　　　　　d. Neurosyphilis.

But clinically it is studied as:
1. PRIMARY SYPHILIS: It usually represents a tissue reaction at the site of entry. It lasts from 3-8 wks.
   It is characterised by the evidence of CHANCRE.
   It is usually a single, painless erosion with an indurated base and clean floor oozing thin serous discharge.
   It is usually found on the genitalia but can be seen affecting the tongue, fingers and lips rarely.
   The regional lymph nodes are bilaterally enlarged. They are discrete, rubbery in consistency and non-tender.
2. SECONDARY SYPHILIS: It can be seen as:
   a. Constitutional Symptoms: Headache, malaise, fever and pain in joints which are worse at Night.
   b. Cutaneous Lesions: The lesions have following characteristics:
      1. They are symmetrical.
      2. Polymorphic lesions.
      3. Non pruritic.
      4. Macular roseola seen commonly on chest and upper arms.
   c. Generalised Lymphadenopathy: All the lymph glands in the order of occipital, epitrochlear, supra trochlear, inguinal, axillary and cervical are enlarged but non tender.
   d. mucous patches: They are white plaques which are easily eroded and leave behind typical SNAIL TRACK ULCERS; Commonly seen in vulva, mouth and prepuce.
   e. Miscellaneous: alopecia, iritis, Hepatitis, arthritis in the form of clutton's joints are seen.
3. TERTIARY SYPHILIS: Clinically it can be divided into
   a. Latent: It is an asymptomatic stage of syphilis in a patient with a definite history revealing the contraction of disease; but exhibiting only a reactive serology.
   b. Late: It is manifested by the appearance of lesions in skin, mucous membranes, bones, joints, tendons and

Skin

viscera with or without cardiovasular and Neurological manifestations.

1. SKIN : The lesions are usually localized and asymmetrical usually infilterated.
2. Mucous membrane: Of the tongue, soft palate lips etc are the sites of affection.
3. Bones: The lesions occur in the form of gummatous ulcers and gumma formation.
4. Visceras: gumma of stomach, liver, spleen are involved.

DIAGNOSIS:
1. PRIMARY STAGE: By Dark ground Illumination Test.
2. SEC AND TERTIARY STAGE: a. VDRL Test.
b. RPR: Rapid plasma Reagen test.
c. C.S.F examination: or colloidal gold Test.

HOMOEOPATHIC MANAGEMENT:

1. AURUM METALLICUM: It is useful in secondary and tertiary stages of syphilis when mentally the patient is very upset with disgust of life and suicidal thoughts constantly prevail throughout.

   It is helpful when the heart is the seat of manifestations. There is constant sensation as if the heart stopped beating for two-three sec followed by a sudden thump.

   All the complaints are worse at night.

2. MERC SOL: It is one of the best suitable remedies when in SECONDARY STAGE there is marked affinity for mucous membranes and the lymphatic system.

   All the complaints are associated with intense weakness.

   There is a general tendency to free perspiration but patient is not relieved by it.

   The glands specially cervical and those of inguinal region are enlarged.

   Complaints usually date back to abuse of mercury and suppression of primary lesions of genitalia.

3. CALOTROPIS: It is good for primary anaemia of syphilis when the patient constantly complains of marked heat in the stomach.

   It is useful in secondary and tertiary stages of syphilis also.

4. CORYDALIS: There are syphilitic affections in the form of ulcers of mouth and fauces. Cachexia is very marked. All the lymph glands are swollen with dry scaly and scabby skin.
5. STILLINGIA: It is useful when the syphilis affects the bones and joints. It is associated with deposits of white sediment in the urine. There is constant aching in the bones of back and extremities. Complaints are worse in afternoon and better in morning.

Q-3. What is Leucoderma? what are the symptoms? Give Homoeopathic Drugs. (1987, 1991 Supp. 1989).

Ans. *LEUCODERMA:* It is an acquired idiopathic depigmentary condition which is characterised by appearance of depigmented macules any and every where on the body.

It affects all the age groups with no predilection to either sex.

ETIOLOGY:

1. Genetic Predisposition
2. Auto Immunity
3. Nutritional: Defects in copper, proteins and vitamins in diet.
4. Endocrines: Thyrotoxicosis and Diabetes mellitus.
5. Infections: ill health, enteric fever, focal sepsis.

CLINICAL FEATURES:

1. AGE AND SEX: There is no predilection for sex but usually affects the persons between 5-20 yrs of age more incidence in extremes of age.
2. MACULES: Depigmented macules with zone of hyperpigmentation appear asymmetrically with predilection for pressure areas like elbows, knees etc.
3. It usually starts and increases in the summer season.

HOMOEOPATHIC DRUGS:

1. ARSENIC SULPH FLAVUM: Clinically it is one of the most useful Remedy. It can be given even when no clinical indications exist.
   Skin is usually chaffed about genitals.

Skin

2. **NITRIC ACID:** It is specially suited to the persons of syphilitic tendency with a H/O mercurial abuse or drug in take. It usually starts from the muco cutaneous junction with constant pricking pains in the affected areas.

   It is associated with splinter like pains in the affected area with VINDICTIVE BEHAVIOUR of the patient.

   All the complaints are usually worse after evening.

3. **SYPHILINUM:** It is suitable to persons of both sycotic and syphilitic tendency who usually suffer from all the complaints at night.

   The lesions are usually reddish brown with a disagreeable odour. The complaints are associated with emaciation.

   The patient has a mania for washing the hands. There is excessive flow of saliva from the mouth, it dribbles away when in sleep.

Q-4. What are the symptoms of Ringworm of groin? Mention 3 best Homoeopathic Remedies (1987).

Ans. The Ringworm affecting the groins is one of the commonest forms of TINEA CRURIS.

It is most prevalent in the summer months caused by the epidermophyton and Trichophyton from infected toes and nails.

SYMPTOMS: 1. Intense itching of the groins is very marked.
2. O/E: Small circinatous patch with mild scaling is seen.

HOMOEOPATHIC REMEDIES:

1. **TELLURIUM:** It is one of the best Remedies used for Ringworm infections. Lesions are ring shaped with offensive odor from affected parts.

   There are foetid exhalations. All the discharges have a fish brine odour.

   The itching is worse at Night, at rest, from friction.

2. **SEPIA:** Herpes circinatus in isolated spots. They usually appear in folds of skin like those of knee and popliteal space. Itching is constant not relieved by scratching.

   Eruptions appear in every spring. The patient is always better by exercise.

3. **BACILLINUM:** It is useful in Ring worm of chronic

nature when the underlying cause is pseudo psora. The skin becomes secondarly infected with eczematisation. The glands of groins are enlarged and tender.

It is usually associated with an increased tendency to hawk the phlegm.

Q-5. What are the symptoms of Herpes Zoster infection? Name 4 drugs to treat post Herpetic Neuralgia. (1982, 1987 Supp).

Ans. Herpes Zoster or shingles is one of the commonest viral infection caused by the H.Z virus or varicella virus.

SYMPTOMS:

1. Onset is sudden with appearance of neuralgic pain, local increased senstivity of the skin.
2. Fever: mild to moderate fever wih marked constitutional symptoms.
3. SKIN LESIONS: There are usually vesicular eruptions appearing along the course of nerves, usually, the single nerve involvement.
4. The vesicles soon become opaque and later may become bullae.
5. The lesion usually disappears leaving behind the temporary pigmentation and faint scarring.
6. The regional glands may be enlarged and painful.

HOMOEOPATHIC TREATMENT:

1. SULPHURIC ACID: The pains are very severe usually (R) sided Neuralgia. The pains are usually severe come and go suddenly with a feeling as if there were subcutaneous ulcer.

   It is good for long lasting effects of trauma and after effects of alcohlism.

   Complaints are better by warmth and lying on affected side.

2. MEZEREUM: The pains are usually severe. They go from inside outside. They are associated with intense chilliness and pruritus.

   The pains are usually of burning nature.

   They are associated with marked senstivity of the affected parts.

Skin

The complaints are worse in cold air, night. Better in open air.

3. SPIGELIA: It is a very good Remedy for (L) sided pains which are very sharp shooting and constantly shifting. They usually involve the zygoma, eyes cheek, teeth and temples.

   Pains are associated with great sensitiveness.
   Complaints are usually worse from touch, motion, noise. But better by lying on (R) side.

4. KALI BICHROMICUM: It is a good Remedy for the post Herpetic neuralgia when the pains are of syphilitic origin.

   The pains are usually of shifting nature and they can be covered with the tip of fingers. It is usually associated with swollen oedomatus uvula.

   The complaints are better from heat; but worse by undressing, beer.

Q-6. What is scabies? suggest the treatment with indications of 4 important drugs with their symptoms. What advice has been given in the organon. (1978 Supp, 1983, 1987 Supp).

Ans. *DEFINITION:* It is a contagious disease caused by the infestation with a mite Sarcoptes Scabei.

The disease is contracted by intimate contact with infected individuals or through infected bed linen or clothing.

SYMPTOMS: 1. Nocturnal pruritus: There is intense itching which is usually worse at Night and in warmth of bed.

2. Fine pin head sized follicular papules with an erythematous base.
3. Excoriations and scratch marks are seen.
4. History of exposure or multiple cases in the family.
5. Burrows traversed by parasites are seen in the interdigital webs, palms, wrists, points of elbow and in periumbilical area.

ADVICE IN ORGANON: Do not use Ext applications. Give a superficial Remedy. But once the acute phase is over give a deep acting constitutional medicine.

TREATMENT:

1. **SULPHUR:** The skin is dry, unhealthy with intense itching and burning. The itching is always worse by scratching and washing.

   Pruritus specially from warmth, in evening, often recurs periodically in spring time and in damp weather. It is associated with redness of the orifices and an empty all gone feeling in stomach.

2. **MERCSOL:** The skin is constantly moist. Excessive perspiration of foul smelling type which does not relieve.

   The pruritus is usually worse at Night. Itching is also aggravated from the warmth of bed.

   The tongue is flabby, moist and large with imprints of teeth; associated with increased Salivation.

3. **SKOOKUM CHUCK:** The skin is dry and irritating. There is intense itching with profuse coryza and sneezing. It is one of the specifics for scabies.

4. **CHRYSAROBINUM:** The scabies when secondarily infected with scabs and crust formation then it should be thought of. There is violent itching of thighs, legs and of ears.

   Dry scaly eruptions with a tendency to form scabs and pus underneath.

Q-7. Name various sexually Transmitted diseases. Name the etiological agents of each and discuss the clinical features of gonorrhoea (1983, 1991).

Ans.
1. Gonorrhoea: - Neisseria Gonorrhoeae.
2. Syphilis-Treponema pallidum.
3. Chancroid-Haemophilus Ducrey.
4. Granuloma venereum-Donovani granulomatis.
5. Lymphogranuloma venerum-Chlamydia.
6. AIDS-HIV VIRUS
7. Genital warts

CLINICAL FEATURES: Gonorrhoea is one of the commonest sexually transmitted diseases caused by Gram-ve Neisseria gonorrhoeae.

Gonorrhea can occur in males, females or even in children and infants.

Skin

CLINICAL MANIFESTATIONS IN A FEMALE:

1. URETHRITIS: The main complaint is dysuria. There is scalding pain when urinating. On examination a yellow purulent discharge can be brought out on masaging.
2. SKENITIS: When the glands are infected a small bead of pus can be expressed by masaging the duct. It can be felt as an indurated mass on the terminal side of urethra.
3. BARTHOLINITIS: The Bartholin's glands lie on the posterior third of each labium majus. The patient complains of a tender swelling or an abscess in the region of vulva. It is usually palpable between the finger and thumb.
4. VULVITIS: The patient complains of pain and swelling. On examination the labia are oedomatous with pus oozing from between the labia minora.
5. CYSTITIS: Due to this patient C/O frequency and urgency in urination. But sometimes strangury with Haematuria is also seen.
6. VAGINITIS: It is very common in the form of discharge per vaginum which is often offensive and sometimes blood stained.
7. CERVICITIS: The patient usually complains of low backache with constant discharge per vaginum. O/E. The cervix is inflammed with swollen lips and evidence of infection is usually seen.
8. PELVIC INFECTION: It usually occurs in the form of fallopian tube blockage, tubo ovarian abscess or sometimes pelvic cellulitis in extremely acute form.

IN A MALE:

1. URETHRITIS: The patient usually complains of scalding pain while urinating. It is associated with urgency of micturition.

There is thick creamy, yellowish green discharge from urethra.

IN THE YOUNG CHILD

1. VULVOVAGINITIS: It is the commonest manifestation in a child. Usually mother notices a white or yellow dis-

charge on the underclothing and the child may or may not give a H/O contact.

IN INFANTS:
1. OPTHALMIA NEONATORUM: There is swelling of eyelids with a purulent discharge. The eyelids are stuck together with the discharge.

Q-8. Differentiate between Ringworm and psoriasis. Describe the treatment of both with the Homoeopathic Remedies. (1985, 1992).

	RING WORM	PSORIASIS
1.	ETIOLOGY: It is a tropical disease caused by the group of fungi like epidermophyton, Trichophyton etc.	It is a Heredo familial disease of unknown etiology.
2.	AGE AND SEX: It usually occurs in middle aged patients of male population.	It can affect the persons of any age or sex.
3.	LESIONS: Are Asymmetrical.	They are bilaterally Symmetrical.
4.	ITCHING: Is very Marked.	No itching.
5.	SITE OF LESION: either in folds, in scalp, or on the whole body.	Predilection for extensor surface of the body and scalp.
6.	WEATHER PREDOMINANCE: more common in summers and rains.	more seen in winters.
7.	COURSE: Is short term with good prognosis.	Course is long term with poor prognosis.
8.	COMPLICATIONS:	Articular

are usually minimal 9. KOEBNER'S PHENOMENON and CANDLE GREASE SIGN are absent.	complications are generally seen. They are usually present.

For Homoeopathic Treatment of Ringworm: See Q-4. and for Psoriasis: See Q-1.

Q-9. Write short notes on:
1. **Alopecia (1988, 1987).**
2. **Dermatitis (1988 Supp)**
3. **Herpes Zoster (1978, 1988 Supp)**
4. **Male pattern Baldness (1987)**
5. **Lichen Planus (1987 Supp)**
6. **Dermal Leishmanoid (1982)**
7. **Leucoderma (1978 D.M.S)**

Ans.

ALOPECIA: Alopecia means hair loss which can be either diffuse or localised in patches.

It is a very common condition in day to day practise.

ETIOLOGY:

Although a definite factor is not known but multiple factors are seen running in the background.
1. Change of climate.
2. Poor diet.
3. Seborrhoea.
4. Pregnancy, delievery.
5. Loss of blood.
6. Mental strains.
7. Typhoid or other febrile illness.

The patterns of alopecia according to the manifestation can be categorised under
a. Cicatrical   b. Non cicatrical.
1. Leprosy   1. Alopecia Areata

2. X-Ray Burn
3. Lupus Vulgaris
2. Tinea
3. Post febrile

TREATMENT: The treatment is according to the underlying cause. But following cares and precautions can be taken in any case of alopecia :--
1. Avoid undue mental strain, trauma or any injurious irradiation.
2. Apply good quality oils and use good shampoos.
3. Do not wash the Hairs too frequently and the hair driers too often.

HOMOEOPATHIC TREATMENT: The drugs like
 a. Lycopodium   b. Fluoric acid
 c. Syphillinum   d. Nat mur   e. phosphorus
can be used.

2. **DERMATITIS:** It can be defined as a non contagious inflammation of the skin characterised by erythema, scaling, oedema, vesiculation and oozing.

ETIOLOGY:
1. Genetic predisposition.
2. Familial Sensitiveness.
3. Personal History of allergy in the form of Hay fever, asthma etc.
4. Psychological factors.

ECZEMATOUS DIATHESIS
SNESITIZERS. ←→ DIET.
IRRITANTS.   TRAUMA.
INFECTIONS.   CLIMATE.
DRUGS.   SEPSIS.
MIND.   NUTRITION.

CLASSIFICATION OF DERMATITIS:
The dermatitis along with eczema, although both are categorically same can be studied under the following heads:
1. Photo Dermatitis
2. Contact Dermatitis
3. Infectious Eczematoid dermatitis
4. Endogenous eczema
5. Infantile eczema

Skin

6. Atopic eczema
7. Nummular Eczema
8. Disseminated Eczema
9. Varicose Eczema
10. Neuro dermatitis
11. Radio dermatitis
12. Dermatitis medicamentosa

TREATMENT:
1. Reassuring he patient and the relatives about the disease.
2. Elimination of predisposing, exciting and complicating causes.
3. Correction of atmospheric temperature.
4. Rest to the affected part.
5. Diet: simple, easily palatable diet with lots of fluids and green leafy vegetables with less of salts, condiments and spices.

3. **HERPES ZOSTER** (1978, 1988 SUPP.)

It is one of the commonest viral infections caused by the Herpes Zoster virus or varicella zoster virus. It is also known as SHINGLES.

ETIOLOGY:
It is caused by the varicella zoalster virus. Physical Injuries, mental trauma, drugs and fevers can act as triggers of the attack.

The virus usually affects the posterior root ganglion.

CLINICAL FEATURES:
1. Onset is sudden with marked constitutional symptoms like malaise, fever, debility and rarely the appearance of rash.
2. Locally it starts with neuralgic pain, increased senstivity of the skin.
3. Moderate fever.
4. Development of Rash in the segmental distribution of the affected nerve root with appearance of Herpetic vesicles on the underlying inflammed bases.

COMPLICATIONS: 1. Post HerpeticNeuralgia.
2. Corneal ulceration.
3. Conjunctivitis.

The above 2 can occur when it involves the branches of TRIGEMINAL NERVE.

TREATMENT:
1. Removal of any underlying cause.
2. Vit B complex therapy should be given.
3. Homoeopathic drugs: like Rhustox, Ran bulbosus, Arsenic album, Dolichos etc can be given.
4. **MALE PATTERN BALDNESS:** (1987.)

It is also called masculine alopecia. It is one of the categories of Idiopathic PREMATURE ALOPECIA.

It exclusively affects the young males. The onset is gradual with receeding hair margin and widening of the forehead, thining of hairs.

ETIOLOGY:
It is usually unknown but a Hereditary cause can always be eliminated.

The distribution of the alopecia is symmetrical. Gradually the hairs become atrophic and lustureless thereby lacking the full growing quality and vigour.

TREATMENT: 1. No definite treatment is known as it is a progressive pattern of baldness with unknown etiology.

But hair transplant or wigs can be tried as a last resort.

5. **LICHEN PLANUS** (1987 SUPP).

It can be defined as an irritating disorder of the skin and mucus membranes characterised by purplish, violet coloured, polyhedral flat topped. itchy papules occuring on the flexor surface and in the mouth.

ETIOLOGY:
Although a definite etiology is unknown but the following have been known to be responsible:
1. Infections: by viruses.
2. Drugs like chloroquinine.
3. Insect bites
4. Physical stresses.

CLINICAL FEATURES:
1. They usually appear as polyhedral firm, purplish vi-

olaceous papules with shiny flat tops.
2. Constant itching is present.
3. The rash is bilaterally symmetrical.
4. SITES: Fronts of wrists, flexor surface of forearm the abdomen, legs, genitalia and the back. There are various varieties of Lichen planus:

1. Annular type: Lichenification following an insect bite.
2. Acute generalised type: Onset is sudden having rash with a short lasting course.
3. Lichen planus verrucus: It occurs as Hyperkeratotic patches on legs.

TREATMENT:
1. Reassurance.
2. Use of some soothing oil or ointment.
3. Homoeopathic Drugs like: Hydrocotyle, Psorinum Radium Bromatum and X-Ray can be used.

6. **DERMAL LEISHMANOID:** (1982).

The skin or cutaneous manifestation of the parasite Leishmania Tropica is called the dermal leishmanoid.

It is also called oriental sore, Delhi boil or Baghdad sore.

The incubation period varies from 1-3 months.

CLINICAL FEATURES:
1. The nodular lesion usually appears on the exposed area of face, cheeks, nose, ears, lips arms and hands.
2. They can be single or multiple, usually they are multiple.
3. Initially the lesion appears as a depigmented macule then becomes nodular and finally ulcerates with a thick crust formation.
4. It is characterised by bluish red infilteration and surrounding Hyperpigmentation.

DIAGNOSIS:
1. Demonstration of L.T bodies in a smear.
2. Culture on N.N.N medium.
3. Biopsy of the Nodule.

7. **LEUCODERMA:** (1978 D.M.S.)

It is an acquired idiopathic depigmentary condition characterised by appearance of depigmented macules of varying sizes and shapes.

ETIOLOGY:
No definite etiology is known.
 But the following causes have been known to occur.
1. NUTRITIONAL: Deficiency of copper, proteins and vitamins in diet.
2. ENDOCRINE: Thyrotoxicosis and diabetes.
3. INFECTIONS: Enteric fever, ill health.
4. DRUGS AND CHEMICALS: Chloroquinine and broad spectrum antibiotics.

CLINICAL FEATURES:
1. The onset is slow and the course is insidious.
2. It appears on the pressure areas like elbows.
3. The asymmetrical distribution of the lesions with Hyperpigmented and ill defined border is characteristic.

PATHOLOGY: There is a defect in enzyme tyrosinase which is held responsible for depigmentation.

TREATMENT:
1. Removal of precipitating factors.
2. Locally application of babchi or croton oil.
3. U. Violet Radiation.
4. Homoeopathic management: The following drugs can be used:
a. Ars sulph flavum.
b. Psorinum
c. Syphilinium
d. Nitric acid
e. Hydrocotyle.

3. LIVER AND GALL BLADDER

Q-1. What are the Symptoms of a patient with viral Hepatitis? Discuss the complications of the disease. Mention it's Homoeopathic treatment. (1981, 1984, 1987 Supp. 1988, 1991 Supp.)

Ans. The invasion of hepatocytes by the viruses of varying etiology leading to clinical manifestations is called viral Hepatitis.

MODE OF ONSET: The following can be seen as the modes:

1. Insidious: With anorexia, gastrointestinal symptoms, low grade fever.
2. Febrile: Temperature rising suddenly to 101°-103°F.
3. Hepatitis without any jaundice.

Clinically the stages can be seen under

PREICTERIC PHASE	ICTERIC PHASE
PRODROMAL PERIOD: 4-7 days	Jaundice appears on 3rd or 4th day
1. Malaise	
2. Anorexia	Urine becomes High Coloured
3. Abdominal distress in the form of fullness or rarely Colic.	Stools are generally pale. Loss of weight. Splenomeagly in few patients.
4. Fever-mild to moderate.	Pruritus ranges from mild to moderate.
5. High Coloured urine.	
6. mild enlargement of liver.	

COMPLICATIONS: If the disease remains undetected or if no treatment is given or inadequate treatment is given, then short lasting self terminating disease can become fatal and may present with any of these complications:
1. Post Hepatitis Syndrome.
2. Relapsing Hepatitis.
3. Cirrhosis.
4. Chronic Hepatitis.
5. Hepatocellular Carcinoma.
6. Cholestatic Hepatitis.
7. Renal failure.

HOMOEOPATHIC TREATMENT:

1. CHELIDONIUM: It is a very efficacious remedy in viral Hepatitis when the patient complains of fullness in the region of liver.

    There is constant dull aching pain in the region of (R) shoulder blade.

    The tongue is yellow coated at the margins with clear base. The patient has great desire for burning hot drinks. All the complaints are better after dinner.

2. PODOPHYLLUM: It is a good remedy when pain with fever is very well marked. There is constant pain in the (R) upper abdomen and the patient constantly rubs and shakes the region of liver with hand.

    The fever paroxysm comes at 7 A.M with chills. The patient is very loquacious during chill but sleeps as soon he starts sweating.

    It is associated with a tendency for loose stools which are generally pale, putrid, painless and profuse.

3. MERC SOL: It is a good remedy for the complaints resulting from mercurial excess or from frequent mercurial preparations.

    There is pain in the region of liver but the patient is unable to lie on (R) side. It is associated with frequent stools passed with tenesmus which is not relieved even after passing stools.

    The patient has marked thirst, despite the fact that the tongue is moist, flabby with the imprints of teeth.

    All the complaints are worse at night.

Liver and Gall Bladder

Q-2. Describe the clinical features, D.D and the management of Amoebiac Hepatitis and liver abscess. (1988 Supp.)

CLINICAL FEATURES

Ans. 1. ONSET: It is usually insidious with no symptoms till the abscess is large.
2. PAIN: Patient constantly complains of dull and aching pain in the region of liver which later on becomes sharp and stabbing.
The pain is usually reffered to the (R) shoulder blade. The pain is increased by deep respiration or by coughing.
3. HEPATO MEAGLY: Localised or generalised enlargement of liver is seen.
4. JAUNDICE: Is usually rare but can be seen.
5. CONSTITUTIONAL SYMPTOMS:
a. High fever with chills and rigors.
b. Emaciation
c. Diffuse joint pains.
6. SYMPTOMS DUE TO EXTENSION:
a. LUNGS: The abscess is coughed up which is usually of choclate colour.
b. PERITONEUM: Presents with pain in abdomen all over with generalised tenderness.

MANAGEMENT:

1. Complete Rest in bed is advisable.
2. Reassurance to the patient and family members.
3. Use of metronidazole in Hepatitis.
4. Aspiration: In liver abscess.
5. Homoeopathic Treatment: Following can be used
a. Chelidonium   b. Sillicea   c. Chenopodium
d. Nat phos e. Myrica.
For D.D. See Q-6.
6. Diet: Simple, low in fats.

Q-3. Describe the cirrhosis of liver. Mention about the management of bleeding because of oesophageal varices. (1988 Supp).

Ans. **CIRRHOSIS** can be defined as a chronic liver disease of diffuse nature, varied etiology and characterised by hepatic cell necrosis, proliferation of connective tissue and regeneration of Nodules

ETIOLOGY:
1. Alcoholism.
2. Infections: Hepatitis B virus infections.
3. Metabolic Diseases.
a. Wilson's Disease.
b. Haemochromatosis.
4. Drugs.

CLINICAL FEATURES:
1. ONSET: Is usually insidious with anorexia, malaise weight loss and loss of libido.
2. HEPATIC SYMPTOMS:
a. Jaundice.
b. Liver palpable in early stages but not in late stages.
3. ASCITES-Shifting Dullness and fluid thrill are positive on examination.
4. CIRCULATORY CHANGES:
a. Spider Telengectasia.
b. Palmer erythema.
c. Cyanosis.
5. PORTAL HYPER TENSION
a. Splenomeagly.
b. collateral vessels.
c. Fetor Hepaticus.
6. ENDOCRINE CHANGES

IN A MALE	FEMALES
1. Gynaecomastia.	Atrophy of Breasts.
2. Atrophy of testis.	Irregular menses.
3. Impotence.	Amenorrhoea.

7. HAEMORRHAGIC TENDENCY:
a. Epistaxis.
b. Menorrhagia.
c. Bruises, purpura.

MANAGEMENT OF OESOPHAGEAL BLEEDING:
1. REST: In bed complete physical and mental.
2. GENERAL MEASURES:
a. Use of blood transfusions.

Liver and Gall Bladder

   b.   Give the Normal saline.
   c.   Give the patient ice cubes to suck.
3.   DRUGS: Drugs like pitressin or somatostatin can be given.
4.   USE OF COMPRESSION TUBE: The sengstaken tube is generally used. It usually has oesophageal and gastric end balloons.

The gastric ballon is inflated. with 20ml of radio opaue dye. The sausage shaped oesophageal ballon is next distended with air.

The tube is pulled up and attached with adhesive tape to the patient's face or suspended over a wheel pulley. It helps in control of bleeding. But it cannot be left for more than 6-7 hrs.

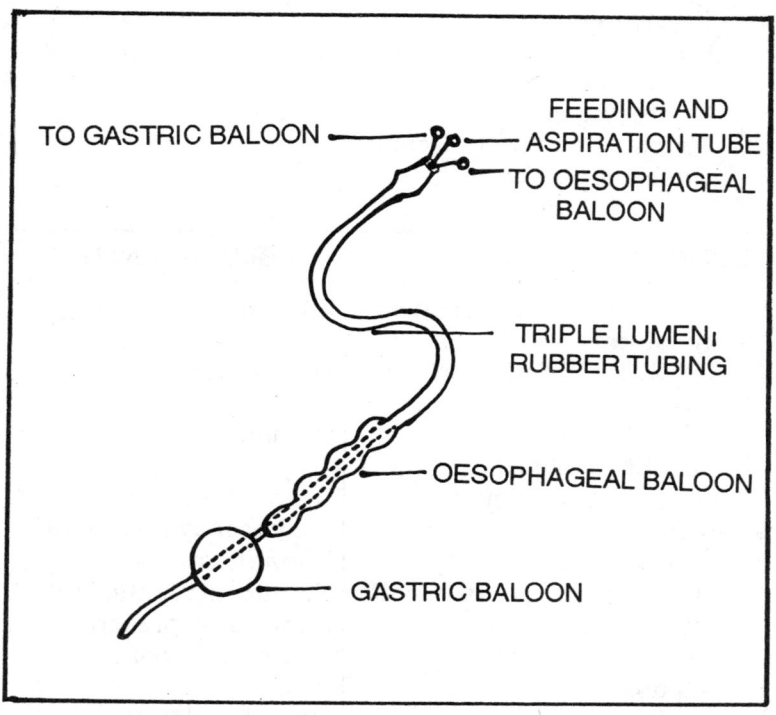

(SENGSTAKEN OESOPHAGEAL TUBE)

5. ENDOSCOPIC SCLEROTHERAPY: In this the varices are sclerosed. It can be either.
   1. Intra variceal 2. Paravariceal
6. SHUNT OPERATIONS: It is usually done in cryptogenic and post necrotic cirrhosis. Porta caval anastomosis or splenorenal shunt is done.

Q-4. What are the common causes of obstructive Jaundice? How would you differentiate it from viral Hepatitis? Mention 4 Homoeopathic Drugs. (1976, 1987).

Ans. CAUSES OF OBSTRUCTIVE JAUNDICE: The jaundice due to obstruction is usually called SURGICAL JAUNDICE.

CAUSES:
1. Gall stones.
2. Foreignbody.
3. Congenital atresia or stricture.
4. CA Head of pancreas.
5. Sclerosing cholangitis.
6. Metastasis in porta Hepatis.
7. Choledochal Cyst.

OBSTRUCTIVE JAUNDICE	VIRAL HEPATITIS
1. ONSET: Is usually sudden and stormy.	It is slow.
2. COLOUR OF SKIN: Yellow, orange or greenish.	Yellow (light)
3. DISTRIBUTION OF PIGMENT: Seen earlier in conjunctiva.	Seen in skin.
4. PRURITUS: Very severe	mild or may be absent.
5. STOOLS: Pale	Normal usually.
6. URINE: B. pigments usually, high coloured urine	No Bile pigments. But Billiribin is present.
7. LIVER: is usually palpable	May or may not be.
8. ANAEMIA: may or may	usually mild.

Liver and Gall Bladder

not be present.	
9. E.S.R: usually (N)	It is raised.
10. VAN DEN BERGH REACTION: Direct Reaction.	Indirect Reaction.
11. PREVIOUS HISTORY: H/O attacks of pain if stone.	H/O exposure to hepatotoxic drugs or contact with other cases of jaundice.
12. LIVER FUNCTION TESTS:	
a. High % of conjugated billirubin.	Raised Conjugated and free billirubin.
b. Raised Alk Phosphatase.	mild increase but usually not raised.

FOR HOMOEOPATHIC TREATMENT SEE Q-1.

FOR OBSTRUCTIVE JAUNDICE

1. CHIONANTHUS: It is a good remedy for obstructive jaundice resulting from gall stones impaction in the common bile duct. The attacks of pain are usually periodical with great nausea and vomiting.
   It is associated with yellowness of conjunctiva with dull frontal headache and listlessness.
   Jaundice is associated with Amenorrhoea.

2. CHOLESTERINUM: It is very good remedy when there is long lasting obstinate engorgement and there is no response to the indicated medicine.
   There is burning pain in the (R) Upper abdomen which constantly hurts the patient. Therefore he walks holding his hand on side.
   Jaundice is usually associated with increased level of cholesterol and opacities of vitreous.

3. CALC CARB: It is specially suitable to the persons of fat, flabby and phlegmatic temprament.
   The patient contantly C/O heaviness and fullness in the region of liver.
   There are frequent sour eructations with sour vomiting. There is complets loss of appetite when over worked.

The bowels are usually constipated and there is profuse sour smelling sweat all over the body. The stools are first hard then pasty then liquid.

All the complaints are usually worse in winters, from moist weather and by exertion.

4. BERBERIS VULGARIS: It is a very good remedy for obstructive jaundice resulting from gall stones impaction. There are sharp stitches in the region of gall bladder.

The pains are sharp, shooting and frequently shifting from one place to another.

There is nausea before breakfast. It is generally associated with urinary disturbances.

The complaints are usually worse from motion and by standing.

Q.5 Define Jaundice, Discuss the indications of chelidonium, Phosphorus, China and Kali Carb. (1975, 1982 Supp, 1982)

Ans JAUNDICE : It is a symptom complex characterised by increase of bile pigments in body fluids and tissues. It is perceptible only when the level of billirubin and it's conjugates exceed 1.5 mg to 2.0mg per 100ml of plasma.

1. CHELIDONIUM : See q-1.
2. PHOSPHORUS : It is particularly useful in Haemato genous jaundice particularly resulting from frequent haemolysis.

It is particularly useful in the persons who are lean, thin with stoop shoulders and thin chest. There is sour taste with sour erutations after every meal.

There is pain in stomach and (r) upper abdomen which is better by cold foods.

Liver is usually congested and palpable with Jaundice. It is generally associated with constipation when the patient passes long slender dog like stools with intense bleeding.

There is great desire for icy cold things, juicy, refreshing things which generally gives relief.

3. CHINA : It is specially suitable to persons who are extremely debilitated specially from loss of vital fluids and nervous erethism.

It it indicated both in Haemolytic and obstructive jaundice when the liver is generally palpable but there is marked sensitiveness to touch.

There are sharp pains in the region of liver which are agg from slightest touch but better on deep pressure. There is flatulence with belching of bitter liquid but it does not give any relief.

The patient usually suffers from painless, nocturnal diarrhoea where stools are frothy, yellow, and contain undigested food.

4. KALI CARB : It is suited to people who are generally fleshy with dropsical and paretic tendencies. The complaints usually result fromthe abuse of mercurial intakes.

There are sharp stitching pains in the region of liver. The patient cannot lie on the (R) side. There is immense flatulence with great desire for sweets.

Pain is associated with nausea which is better lying down. Anxiety felt in stomach with constant full feeling.

The stools are usually large, with stitching pains sometime before passing stools.

The complaints are usually worse early morning.

It is associated with marked sweatiness, backache and prostration.

Q.6. What is liver abscess? Discuss the D. D., Complications and general management. (1992).

Ans. It can be defined as the commonest complications of Amoebiasis which is usually characterised by presence of single abscess in the postero superior surface of the Right lobe.

DIFFERENTIAL DIAGNOSIS

1. VIRAL HEPATITIS : It is a viral infestation of hepatoytes. The course is usually short lasting. It is associated with mild to moderate fever with pain and tenderness on palpation and JAUNDICE.
   The LFT are usually diagnostic
2. AUTE CHOLE CYSTITIS : The patient usually a female of fat, flabby diathesis complains of attacks of severe pain in the region of liver. The pain is often reffered to the tip of the shoulder. It is generally associated with

Jaundice and constipaton. On examination the patient gives Toxic look; with tenderness on palpation.
3. HYDATID CYST : There is infestation of liver cells by the Echinococus granulosus. There is generally a H/o contacts with dogs. Although no definite features but Casonis Test is +ve.
4. SUBAUTE BACTERIAL ENDOCARDITIS : It is generally seen in patients with a previous H/o valvular heart disease. The characterstic feature is the presence of Haemic murmurs, Haematuria, splinter Haemorhages in the Nail bed with splenomeagly. The E.S.R. is raised.

Q.7 Give the treatment of portal cirrhosis (1974 D.M.S. west Bengal, 1975).
Ans The treatment can be discussed under :
1. **GENERAL MANAGEMENT :**
A. REST : In bed is very essential.
B. DIET : Low fat intake with less salt. Total calories of 2000 Kcal should be given.
C. REMOVAL OF ANY KNOWN CAUSE :
D. ABSTINENCE : from alcohol completely is essential.

HOMOEOPATHIC MANAGEMENT :
1. MERC SOL : See q-1 under Homoeopathic Treatment.
2. PODOPHYLLUM ; See q-1
3. NASTURTIUM : It is generally indicated in cases with dropsy. Constipation is usually associated with excessive desire to sleep and general weakness.
4. SULPHURIC ACID : It is one of the best remedies for cirrhosis resulting from excessive intake of alcohol. There is generally a familial tendency to take alcohol. There is relaxed feeling in stomach with sour eructations which even sets teeth on edge.

The pain in the region of liver is associated with bleeding from oesophageal varices.

There are severe pains in the region of liver with flushes of heat, tremors and weakness.

The complaints are better by lying on the affected side and from warmth.

Liver and Gall Bladder

Q-8 What are the important causes of irregular enlargement of liver? Give the Differential Diagnosis (1982 Supp.)

Ans The irregular enlargement of liver due to varying etiology can be classified with or without Jaundice.

WITH JAUNDICE	WITH JAUNDICE
1. Hepatic Cirrhosis	1. Gumma
2. Late Secondary Tumours	2. Secondary Tumours
3. Cholangio Heaptic adenoma.	3. Polycystic disease.

DIFFERENTIAL DIAGNOSIS :

1. CONGENITAL : Riedle's Lobe. It is usually palpable on the (L) side of the midine. It is generally asymptomatic.
2. HYDATID CYST : It is generally soft to firm in consistency. The liver is palpable with a positive CASONIS TEST.
3. CONGESTIVE HEPATOMEAGLY : Seen in C.C.F., portal Hypertension
   The liver is usually uniformly enlarged and soft in consistency. Due to excesive circulation the venous hum can be heard over it.
4. BILLIARY OBSTRUCTION : By gall stones, CA Head of pancreas.
   The liver is usually regularly enlaged with a FIRM CONSISTENCY on palpation. Beside this, the gall bladder may also be palpable.
5. MYELOID METAPLASIA : Seen in multiple myeloma, secondary carcinoma of bone, Leukemia etc.
   The liver usually shows a regualr enlargement But the diagnosis is generally made by the respective blood picture and by the IMMUNOGRAM; showing relative activity of IgA, IgG, IgM etc.

Q.9 Write short notes on :
1. **Hydatid cyst of liver (1988 supp)**
2. **Hepatomeagly (1984)**
3. **Signs of chronic liver failure (1989)**
4. **S. Billirubin and its Importance (1987 Supp).**
5. **Nut meg liver (1976)**

6. Hob Nail liver (1977)
7. Billiary Cirrhosis (1981)
8. vanden Burgh Reaction (1982 Supp.)
9. Compare Hepatitis A and B (1991.)
10. Australia Antigen (1988 Supp.)

Ans. 1. **HYDATID CYST OF LIVER :** It is a parasitic infestation by ECHINOCOCUS GRANULOSUS.

It is usually transmitted by the contact of dogs either directly or by allowing the dog to feed from the same dish or by taking uncooked vegetables contaminated with infected faeces.

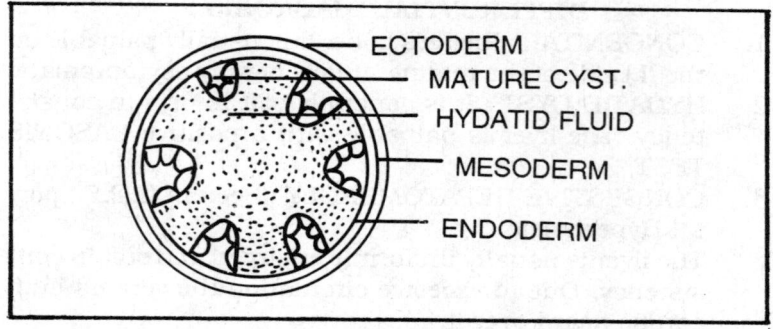

(HYDATID CYST.)

SYMPTOMS AND SIGNS :
1. ASYMPTOMATIC : It usually remains asymptomatic unless secondary infection takes place.
2. HEPATOMEAGLY : There is painless enlargement of liver.
3. FEVER : when it gets secondary infected fever results.
4. JAUNDICE : Due to pressure on bile ducts.
5. CONSTITUTIONAL UPSETS WITH TOXAEMIA : may occur if it ruptures.

DIAGNOSIS :
1. Ultrasound of liver.
2. Casoni's Test.

2. **HEPATOMEAGLY :** When the liver is enlarged and palpble per abdomen it is called hepatomeagly.

Liver and Gall Bladder

ETIOLOGY :

1. Infections : viral hepatitis, infectious mononucleosis, syphilis, Amoebiasis, malaria, Kala azar.
2. Toxic causes : Drugs like chloroquinine, carbon tetra chloride
3. Degenerative : Fatty degeneration.
4. Tumours and cysts : Hepatoma, metastatic tumours.
5. Congenital : Riedle's lobe
6. Billiary obstrution : Gall stones, stricture or atrophy of bile ducts.
7. Congestive Causes : C.C.F, Constrictive pericarditis, portal hypertension.

CLINICALLY SIGNIFICANT POINTS TO ASSESS HEPATOMEAGLY.

1. The liver should be palpated very gently by asking the patient to lie down and take deep breaths.

   The Hand in a vertical position should be kept facing the epigastrium; and it should be moved gradually to feel the liver moving against the chest movements.

2. The consistency : usually in acute and congestive conditions the liver is soft to firm in consistency and painful.

   But in chronic conditions it is firm to hard in consisitency and painless.

3. **SIGNS OF CHRONIC LIVER FAILURE :**

   Hepatocellualr failure can complicate almost all forms of liver disease and may be precipitated by infections, surgical operation, or some drugs.

GENERAL FEATURES :

1. Weakness and general failure of health.
2. Hyper dynamic circulation manifested by flushed extremities, bounding pulse.
3. Fever is common
4. Septicaemia in terminal stages.
5. Foetar hepaticus.

PARTICULAR FEATURES :

A. ENDOCRINE
1. Loss of libido

2. Hair loss
3. In males
a. Gynaecomastia
b. Testiular atrophy
c. Impotence
4. In females :
a Amenorrhoea
b. Irregular menses
c. Breast atrophy.
B. JAUNDICE
C. HAEMORRHAGIC TENDENCY :
1. Bruises
2. Epistaxis
3. Menorrhagia
D. FEATURES OF PORTAL HYPERTENSION
1. Splenomeagly
2. Collateral circulatory channels are established.
E. ASCITES.

4. **SERUM BILLIRUBIN AND ITS IMPORTANCE :**

Billirubin is a metabolic product of the breakdown of R.B.C. It is usually yellow in colour and therefore stains the tisues also yellow.

It is generally found in two forms

1. Conjugated : Conjugated billirubin is water soluble and cannot cross the small bowel but is excreted in the urine and makes it dark.
2. Unconjugated : Billirubin is lipid souluble and can cross the bowel wall from blood. It does not cross the Renal glomerulus and therfore prduces ACHOLURIC JAUNDICE.

Total Billirubin should be more than 70 μ mol/l to produce JAUNDICE CLINICALLY.

IMPORTANCE

1. It is considered to be one of the best known markers of LIVER FUNCTION TESTS.
2. The estimation of Billirubin by van den bergh's reaction will help to know the type of Jaundice whether Haemolytic, heaptic or obstructive type.
3. It helps in knowing the extent of liver damage.

Liver and Gall Bladder

5. **NUTMEG LIVER :** Chronic passive congestion of liver resulting from (r) heart failure produces typical appearance of congestive red accentuation centrally of liver cells histologically.

HISTOPATHOLOGICAL CHANGES :
1. The liver lobules show congestive red accentation in the centre with a pale periphery.
2. Widening of space of disse is usually seen.
3. Central veins and central portions of vasular sinusoids show enlargement.

6. **HOB NAIL LIVER :** The characteristic histological changes occuring in the liver cells due to alcohol or in fatty degeneration leading to PORTAL CIRRHOSIS is called Hob nail liver.

On palpation the surface is usually irregular and uneven; due to formation of multiple nodules.

HISTOLOGICAL CHANGES :
1. Swelling and Necrosis of scatttered hepatocytes.
2. Neutrophillic reaction in and about the foci of Necrosis.
3. The presence of Hyaline bodies.
4. Diffuse fibrosis around the liver lobules and also the central veins leading to the formation of micro and macro nodules.

7. **BILLIARY CIRRHOSIS :** It is one of the types of cirrhosis resulting from prolonged obstruction any where between bile ducts and the papilla of vater.

TYPES :
1. PRIMARY BILLIARY CIRRHOSIS : It predominately affects the females in the middle age group.
2. SYMPTOMS
a. Pruritus is the commonest complaint.
b. Jaundice is also present.
c. Diarrhoea resulting from mal abosorption of fat is generally seen.
d. Bone pain or fractures are common.
e. Neurological : Pain and tingling in hands and feet due to lipid infilteration.

f. Xanthomas are seen.
g. O/E : spleen and liver are palpable.

SECONDARY BILLIARY CIRRHOSIS: It develops due to prolonged obstruction of bile ducts either by gall stones. strictures or by sclerosing cholangitis.

SYMPTOMS AND SIGNS :
1. Features of underlying causes like pain, fever, Jaundice are present.
2. Finger clubbing is common.
3. Xanthomas are generally seen.

8. **VANDEN BERGH REACTION :**

It is one of the tests to assess the Liver Functioning. It is helpful in both the obstructive type and Hepatic type of Jaundice.

TYPES : It is usually of 2 types :
1. DIRECT REACTION : Add 1ml of reagent to 1ml of serum : 3 types of reactions are seen
a. Immediate : A violet colour due to formation of diazo billrubin in 10-30 seconds.
b. Delayed : No change in appearance for 5-15min. then reddish colour develops which gradually becomes violet
c. Biphasic : A red colour appears promptly but takes a longer time to change to violet.
2. INDIRECT : It is essential to determine S. Billirubin quantitatively. 1ml of serum is mixed with 2ml of 95% alcohol. After shaking or centrifuging, to 1ml of supernatant fluid and 0.25 ml of the Reagent add 0.5ml of alcohol. A reddish violet colour develops immediately.

INTERPRETATION :
1. Prompt direct Reaction - In obstructive Jaundice.
2. Indirect Delayed Direct - Haemolytic Jaundice.
3. Direct Reaction - Hepatic Jaundice.

SOLUTION USED :
1. Conc Hcl 15ml, Sulphanillic acid 1gm with 100 ml distilled water.
2. sodium nitrite 0.5gm with 1000ml of distilled water.

Liver and Gall Bladder

9. **COMPARE HEPATITIS A AND B :**

HEPATITIS A	HEPATITIS B
1. ONSET : abrupt and often febrile.	Insidious usually afebrile.
2. INCUBATION PERIOD : About 5-50 days	It is about 50-150 days.
3. AGE : usually children and young adults.	Any age can be affected
4. ROUTE : Oro faecal route	By blood, intimate personal contact or sexual inter-course.
5. DURATION OF JAUNDICE : shorter	Is generally longer
6. INFECTION OF CONTACTS may occur.	They do not occur
7. ABNORMAL LFT : preceedes by symptoms for several days.	often precede symptoms for several days.
8. CARRIER STAGE : Not seen.	It is commonly found
8. MORTALITY : is low	is very high.
10. HB Ag IN BLOOD : less often found.	is generally present.
11. PROPHYLACTIC VALUE OF GAMMA GLOBULINS is good	is doubtful

10. **AUSTRALIA ANTIGEN :** The surface antigen HBSAG found in the blood of the persons suffering from Hepatitis B is called Australia antigen.

It is so called because it was first found in the serum of Australian Aborigine by Dr Blumberg.

HBSAG or Australia antigen is one of the most significant markers of Hepatitis B infection clinically.

It is generally produced in abundance by the infected liver cells.

DIMENSIONS : In the serum it is seen as a spherical suspension measuring 22mm in diameter. It is long, tubular and filamentous.

It is generally found free in the circulation.

It can be detected as early as 1 week after the infection. But the level is generally undetectable 3 months after the exposure.

4. BONES AND JOINTS

Q-1. What are the main features of Ankylosing Spondylitis? Mention the conditions you would like to consider as Differential Diagnosis. What are the 4 main drugs used in it's treatment. (1987, 1988.)

Ans. It is one of the commonest forms of (SSA) Sero Negative spondarthrides which is characterised by the chronic inflammation of the joints of spine and sacroliac joints with stiffening and fusion of the axial skeleton.

CLINICAL FEATURES:
1. It is exclusively found in males (M:F 4:1) of the 2nd to 3rd decade.
2. ONSET: is generally insidious with low back ache or stiffness in the low back which is generally neglected by the patient.
3. Gradually it increases and involves the spine in a direction from below upwards with increasing pain and stiffness.
4. It usually involves the S.I joints but in later stages costochondral, costovertebral and sterno clavicular joints are involved with fixation of chest wall and scapulae.
5. After a period of years whole spine is involved giving rise to what is called POKER'S BACK.
6. ASSOCIATED COMPLAINTS:
a. Achilles Tendinitis.
b. Plantar Fascitis.
c. Fixation of chest with complete absence of chest expansion.
d. Kyphosis may develop.
e. Keratitis and uveitis may also be seen.

SIGNS:
1. Shober's test is positive.
2. Pain is elicited by pelvic compression test, and pump handle test.

DIFFERENTIAL DIAGNOSIS
1. RADOLOGICAL: Endemic Flurosis.
2. FROM LOW BACKACHE
a. O.A of spine.
b. Lumbo sciatica syndrome.
c. Fibrositis.
d. Spondylolisthesis.

HOMOEOPATHIC DRUGS:
1. ARNICA: It is specially suited to those persons who are easily affected by any trauma.

   The joints of spine are usually very painful to touch. Patient will not allow anyone to touch them or even approach them.

   It is good for ascending type of Rheumatism when pain is of sore bruised type with constant aching. There is Hardness of the bed with a feeling as if everything is sore and hard when lying over it.

   The complaints are worse from least touch, by motion but better by rest with head low.

2. RHUSTOX: It is a very good remedy for affection of joints when the complaints are worse from exposure to damp weather or from cold.

   There are tearing pains in tendons, ligaments and in fasciae. The rheumatic pains are constantly shifting but better by motion.

   There is pain and stiffness in small of back better by lying on something hard.

3. STRYCHNINUM: It is a good remedy for Rheumatic stiffness with Cramp like pains. The pains are generally associated with violent jerking, twitching and trembling. The spasms are provoked by slightest touch and attempt to move.

   It is generally associated with marked irritability.

   The pain is better by lying on the back.

Bones and Joints

4. MEDORHINUM: It is one of the efficient Nosodes used in chronic Rheumatism of the back. It is generally given on a SYCOTIC BACKGROUND.

There is intense prostration with constant pain in lower back. The backache is better by profuse urination.

Heels and balls of feet feel tender. The complaints are generally worse when thinking of them and better when at sea shores or lying on stomach and in damp weather.

Q-2. Discuss Gout. Mention its signs and Symptoms. Give the Differential diagnosis. Mention 4 Homoeopathic Drugs
(1977, 1981, Supp, 1987, 1988 Supp, 1989.)

Ans. GOUT: can be defined as a disorder of purine metabolism resulting in Hyperuricaemia and deposition of urate Crystals in the Synovium; and clinically manifesting as recurrent acute arthritis progressing to chronic deforming arthritis, formation of tophi with development of Systemic complications.

ETIOLOGY:
1. Primary or genetic: It accounts for 95% of the total cases.
2. SECONDARY: It can be either due to diminished excretion of Uric acid or due to increased production.
a. DUE TO DIMINISHED EXCRETION
1. Renal failure.
2. myxoedema
3. Drugs
4. Down's Syndrome
b. DUE TO INCREASED PRODUCTION
1. Psoriasis
2. Leukemia
3. Polycythaemia vera.

CLINICAL FEATURES:
1. Asymptomatic: It usually manifests as Hyperuricemia.
2. **ACUTE GOUT :**
a. Onset is sudden generally in the middle of Night.
b. Temperature is usually 101-102°F and after a bout of sweating patient may go to sleep.

c.   on waking he finds the joint is hot, swollen and tender. It is so painful that he does not allow it to touch.
d.   The pain ceases in day time but becomes worse following night.
e.   It exfoliates mildly leaving no residual signs.
3.   **CHRONIC GOUT**
a.   The patient is generally over middle age with a frequent H/O acute or subaute attacks.
b.   It may present as dyspepsia, phlebitis or even as H.T or Secondary O.A of Knee.

SIGNS ON EXAMINATION:
1.   Gouty Tophi in ear lobes, in the arms or along the cartilages.
2.   PALSTERER'S HAND: White striae or lines appear along the lines of palmer creases of hands.

The attack is generally precipitated by:
1.   Alcohol.
2.   Obesity.
3.   Local injury.
4.   Following some infection.
5.   Vit B_{12} deficiency.

DIFFERENTIAL DIAGNOSIS:
1.   Acute Rheumatism.
2.   Degenerative arthritis with acute Inflammation.
3.   Acute calcific tendinitis.
4.   Haematoma.
5.   Subacute Bacterial Endocarditis (SABE) with Suppurative arthritis.
6.   Psoriatic Arthritis.
7.   Inflamed Bunions.

HOMOEOPATHIC DRUGS
1.   GUAIACUM: It is specially adapted to the persons of arthritic, rheumatic and Tonsillitic diathesis. Rheumatic pains in feet with pricking sensation.

A feeling of heat in the affected limbs is highly characteristic. Gouty and Rheumatic pain in head and face extending to neck.

The complaints are generally associated with unclean odour from whole body.

Bones and Joints

The pains are worse from motion, heat and cold wet weather Better by external pressure.

2. OXALIC ACID: It is specially suited to the persons of uric acid diathesis who constantly pass urates in the urine.

There are sharp, shooting pains in the big toe which are sharp electric shock like with shifting nature. They are associated with numbness and an increased tendency to pass urates in the urine with oxalates.

The complaints are generally worse on (L) side, from slightest touch and by shaving and when thinking of his ailments.

3. URTICA URENS: When Rheumatism is associated with urticaria like eruptions then it should be thought of.

The symptoms usually return at the same time of year.

It also antidotes ill effects of crabs. The pains are generally worse from snowair, cool moist air and by touch.

4. THUJA OCCIDENTALIS: It is a remedy suitable to the persons of Sycotic diathesis. There are constant aching pains in the affected joint which are usually worse early morning. When walking limbs feel as if made of wood or glass and would break easily. Pain in heels and tendoachilles.

The pains are worse at 3 A.M and 3 P.M. from cold damp air but feels relieved by drawing up the limbs.

Q-3. Discuss the clinical features of Rheumatoid Arthritis. How would you differentiate it from osteoArthritis? Mention it's treatment and homoeopathic medicines (1978, 1980, 1985, 1985 Supp. 1992.)

Ans. RHEUMATOID ARTHRITIS: It is one of the commonest chronic seropositive inflammatory joint disease characterised by symmetrical involvement of the small joints.

ETIOLOGY:

Although a definite etiology is not known but following features play an important role.

1. AGE: usually occurs in 3rd decade of life and onwards.

2. SEX: more common in females.
3. CLIMATE: It is a disease of temperate climate.
4. FAMILY HISTORY: Patients with a family history of disease have increased frequency of HLA antigen DR_4.
5. PSYCHOLOGICAL FACTORS: preceeding psychical or emotional shock is common.
6. TRAUMA: It may start in a joint which has been the seat of trauma.

CLINICAL FEATURES:

1. ONSET: It can be either dramatic with marked constitutional symptoms or it can be insidious with involvement of one or more joints.
2. CONSTITUTIONAL SYMPTOMS: like undue fatigue, weight loss, poor appetite, general malaise and fever are present.
3. PAIN AND STIFFNESS: in the affected joints is seen. The pain is experienced on moving the joint and stiffness is felt early morning which is relieved after walking.
4. SIGNS ON EXAMINATION:
   1. Spindle shaped swelling of Proximal I.P joints.
   2. Swan Neck Deformity: Where there is flexion at Distal I.P joint and extension at prox I.P JOINT.
   3. BOUTINORRERE'S DEFORMITY: It is the reverse of Swan Neck deformity.
   4. ZLINE OR HITCH HIKER'S THUMB:
   5. DROPPED FINGERS
   6. SUBLUXATION: of Knee.
   7. Hammer Toes
   8. Hallux Valgus: Lateral deviation of big toe.

TREATMENT:

1. In acute cases rest in bed.
2. Use of Splints.
3. Use of Anti Inflammatory drugs.
4. Physiotherapy is required.

HOMOEOPATHIC MANAGEMENT:

1. ACTACEA SPICATA: Sharp Rheumatic pains in small joints, wrist ankles and toes. Swelling of joints from slightest fatigue.

The wrist is swollen, red and is worse by any motion. There is sudden lassitude after talking or eating.

2. **VIOLA ODORATA**: It is a good remedy for Rheumatism of the small joints specially with a pressing pain in (R) carpal and metacarpal joint.

   It is associated with milky urine which smells strong. The complaints are worse from cool air.

3. **PULSATILLA**: It is a good remedy for arthritis of the small joints when pains are sharp and constantly shifting and changing place from one to another. The pain is associated with chilliness. They are better by motion and in open air.

4. **CAULOPHYLLUM**: It is one of the best remedies for small joint affections when there are sharp needle like pricking pains which constantly shift from one place to another.

   There are cutting pains on closing the hands. In females, it may be associated with Rigid os and severe pains during menses.

   All the complaints are made worse from motion.

RHEUMATOID ARTHRITIS	**OSTEOARTHRITIS**
1. ONSET: usually acute to subacute.	Insideous.
2. AGE: Between 20-40 yrs.	Above 40 yrs.
3. GENERAL CONDITION: is under nourished.	Patient is well nourished.
4. JOINTS: They are symmetrical and generalised Proximal I.P Joints.	usually weight bearing joints of Knee, spine are involved.
5. E.S.R: moderately raised.	Not raised.
6. NATURE: It is an atrophic type of arthritis.	It is a Hypertrophic type of arthritis.
7. HEBREDEN'S NODES: absent.	They are Present in Primary O.A.
8. SYNOVIAL FLUID: is Inflammatory.	It is non inflammatory
9. R.A FACTOR: +ve	is -ve.

Q-4. Discuss the role of Pyrogenum in a case of PYOGENIC ARTHRITIS and suggest the Homoeopathic Treatment (1982.)

Ans. PYROGENUM: It is a nosode obtained from the lean beef.

It is a great remedy for SEPTIC STATES with intense restlessness.

The arthritis of pyogenic origin needs a special mention when the pains are of burning nature with complete intolerance of them.

The pains are associated with chilliness and High temperature. But the pulse is generally disproportionate with the degree of fever.

All the discharges are highly offensive with great restlessness and inability to lie on the bed because it feels very hard.

The tongue is red and clean as if varnished. There is relief from motion.

HOMOEOPATHIC TREATMENT:
1. STRYCHNINUM: See Q-1
2. ARNICA: See Q-1
3. RHUSTOX See Q-1

Q-5. Discuss the Differential diagnosis and management of Red painful swollen Knee joint in a 6yrs old child (1989, 1991 Supp.)

Ans. 1. RHEUMATIC ARTHRITIS: It usually follows an attack of streptococcal infection. There are sharp wandering pains with marked constitutional features.

The presence of raised E.S.R and ASO titre and Creative protein is diagnostic.

2. HAEMOARTHROSIS: It is generally seen in the cases of Haemophillia when there is bleeding in the joint. There is generally a previous H/O purpura, epistaxis or bruises.

It generally follows minor trauma. Bleeding and clotting time should be checked for.

3. HENOCH SCHLOEIN PURPURA: It usually presents with a catabolic effect. The joints are swollen with

Bones and Joints

erythematous rash all over the body specially on abdomen with marked constitutional symptoms. Sometimes the visceral catastrophe in the form of internal bleeding may occur.
4. OSTEO MYELITIS NEAR KNEE JOINT: Young child usually presents with fever. There is pain around the affected joint with intense swelling and sequesterum formation.

There is raised E.S.R with polymorpho Nuclear Leucolytosis.
5. SUPRAPATELLAR ABSCESS: There is fever with chills and rigors. The joint is extremely tender with complete avoidance of being touched.
6. LEUKAEMIA: It is usually seen as the acute exacerbation of this chronic myeloid metaplasia.

It is generally associated with splenomeagly, lymph adenopathy and History of recurrent infections.
7. STILL'S DISEASE: It is generally seen affecting the single joint with marked constitutional symptoms.

MANAGEMENT:
1. Rest in bed.
2. Splinting of the joint.
3. Use of Anti-inflammatory drugs.
4. Removal of any underlying cause of the pathology
5. Homoeopathic Drugs like: Belladona, Pyrogenum, sillicea, viola odorata can be used.

Q-6. Discuss the etiopathogenesis of cervical spondylosis with clinical features and treatment. (1991)

Ans. It can be defined as a disease of usually unknown etiology which is characterised by the degenerative changes in the cervical vertebrae with gradual reduction of joint space.

ETIOLOGY:
1. Age Between 60-70 yrs.
2. Sex: Both sexes are affected equally.
3. Trauma: It may act as a precipitating factor.

CLINICAL FEATURES:

1. **ONSET**: Is usually gradual with pain and restriction of movements in the region of neck but ocasionally it can be dramatic.
2. The following group of clinical presentations can be seen.

a. RADICULAR SYMPTOMS: They are due to compression of one or more nerve roots.

There is severe pain in the neck which is reffered to the distribution of compressed nerve.

Neck is rigid and held in flexion.

b. CORD COMPRESSION DUE TO CERVICAL MYELOPATHY:

There is dysthesia in the hands, weakness and clumsiness of the hands and spastic weakness of the lower limb. There is combination of diminution of some tendon reflexes with exaggeration of others.

c. PAIN: Acute disc protrusion is associated with severe pain, muscular spasm and rigidity of neck muscles.
d. HEADACHE: The pain is in the base of brain and often spreads upwards from the back of the head to the frontal region. It is usually worse in morning.
e. VERTIGO: The flexion or rotation of neck may precipitate the attacks of giddiness; due to Compression of vertebral arteries.

TREATMENT:

1. Rest in bed in acute stages.
2. Use of analgesic in acute painful stage.
3. Neck collar can be used.
4. In the long run the neck exercises are done with or without traction.
5. Homoeopathic Treatment: Drugs like causticum, calc Fluor, medorrhinum, Lachnanthes can be used.

Q-7. Compare Rheumatic Arthritis with Rheumatoid Arthritis (1991.)

Ans. RHEUMATIC ARTHRITIS	RHEUMATOID ARTHRITIS
1. ONSET: is always	It is gradual but

Bones and Joints

RHEUMATIC ARTHRITIS	RHEUMATOID ARTHRITIS
sudden and dramatic.	ocasionally dramatic.
2. AGE/SEX: It is seen in the children and young people of age group 5-15 yrs. Both the sexes are equally affected.	It occurs in the females of middle age group from 30-40 yrs.
3. JOINTS INVOLVED: It involves multiple joints at a time.	It involves symmetrically the proximal I.P. joints.
4. PAINS: arc of wandering type, going from one joint to another.	It is constant.
5. PAST HISTORY: H/O sore throat or streptococcal infections.	No such history.
6. DIAGNOSTIC TEST: Aso titre, C.Reative protein are +ve.	R.A factor is +ve.

Q-8. Describe the etiology, pathology and signs of Arthritis of Knee. Describe the management of such a case. (1977 Supp.)

Ans. ARTHRITIS OF KNEE: It is generally a degenerative condition of the joint which is progressive in character. It is an age related disease and therefore starts after the age of 45 yrs.

ETIOLOGY

1. Age: It is an age related degenerative disorder.
2. Sex: Incidence is equal in both sexes.
3. Secondary causes:
a. Trauma.
b. Chondrocalcinosis.
c. Systemic Lupus Erythematosus.
d. Gout.
e. R.A.

CLINICAL FEATURES:
SYMPTOMS:
1. Pain in the knee joint which is generally worse at rest or at first motion but better by continous motion.
2. STIFFNESS: Patient Complaints of heaviness with a contracted feeling in the joint felt early morning on waking up.
3. GRATING SOUNDS: In the joint on motion.

SIGNS
1. The joint is swollen.
2. On palpation grunting or crepitations can be heard.
3. Radiological Signs:
a. marked prominence of Tibial tuberosity.
b. Reduction of joint space with destruction of articular cartilage.
c. Presence of osteophytes.

TREATMENT:
1. Physiotherapy with diathermy is useful.
2. Use of analgesics in severe pain.
3. Homoeopathic management: Drugs like Bryonia, Rhustox, O.A nosode, Caustium can be used.

Q-9. Write short Notes on
1. **Diagnosis of R.A affecting the knee joint (1987 Supp.)**
2. **Homoeopathic Treatment of Gout (1991 Supp.)**
3. **Charcot's Joints (1974 Supp.)**
4. **Osler's Nodes (1977.)**

Ans. 1. DIAGNOSIS OF RA AFFECTING THE KNEE JOINT:
1. History of affection of other joints in the body symmetrically.
2. R.A factor +ve
3. E.S.R is raised
4. Presence of Antinuclear Antibodies in the Serum.
2. **HOMOEOPATHIC TREATMENT OF GOUT:**
See Q-2.
3. **CHARCOT'S JOINTS:** They are one of the forms of

Bones and Joints

TROPHIC CHANGES affecting the joints.

The joints are usually painless with indurated margin and the depth is upto the bone.

The Knee and Hip joints are commonly affected. The affected joints become disorganised and there is enormous effusion in the joint. The ends of the bones forming the joint with periarticular tissues are all washed.

The characteristic features are
1. Complete absence of pain.
2. Increased range of movement.
3. Easy dislocation of the joint.
4. **OSLER'S NODES:** They are semitender nodules varying from 0.5 to 1.5 cm in diameter.

They are seen on the palmar and plantar aspects of finger and toe tips caused by the minute emboli of the cutaneous superficial Terminal vessels; or by arteritis of smaller vessels with immune complex deposition.

They are diagnostic of SUB ACUTE BACTERIAL ENDO-CARDITIS.

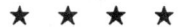

5. EXCRETORY SYSTEM

Q-1. Describe the polycystic diseases of Kidney and it's complications (1988.)

Ans. This is one the commonest congenital abnormalities of the Kidneys which is characterised by the development of multiple cysts in the parenchyma of the Kidneys. It is an autosomal dominant condition

ETIOLOGY:
1. AGE AND SEX: It can be seen in any age group but becomes manifest clinically only in the 4th or 5th decades of life.
The sex incidence is equal.
2. ANAMOLIES ASSOCIATED: Anamolies like spina bifida, cryptorchidism are usually associated.

PATHOLOGY: The Kidneys become enormously enlarged. The surface gives the appearance of many bubbles. The cysts of varying sizes some containing clear cystic fluid, some blood and some with coagulated fluid are seen.

CLINICAL FEATURES:
1. RENAL ENLARGEMENT: The kidneys are palpable per abdomen on routine examination.
2. PAIN: There is constant, dull aching pain in the region of kidneys very rarely it may take the form of Renal colic.
3. HAEMATURIA: Due to over distension the cysts rupture and give rise to bloody urine.
4. SIGNS OF INFECTION: Pyelonephritis usually takes place in neglected cases.
5. URINARY DISTURBANCES:
a. Patient passes abundant quantities of low specific

gravity urine.
b. Urine contains trace of albumin.
6. HYPERTENSION: When a patient in middle age presents with hypertension, then it should be ruled out.
7. URAEMIA: In later stages anorexia, headache and gastric symptoms may be predominent indicating renal failure.

DIAGNOSIS: By excretory urography.

COMPLICATIONS OF POLYCYSTIC KIDNEY DISEASE:
1. Persistent Hypertension.
2. Renal Failure.
3. Interestitial Nephritis.
4. Persistent Haematuria.
5. Rupture of Kidneys.
6. Pressure symptoms on associated organs.

Q-2. What is PyeloNephritis? How would you establish the diagnosis? Give it's detailed management. (1988 Supp.)

Ans. **PYELONEPHRITIS:** It is a form of chronic interestitial nephritis resulting from recurrent urinary tract infections.

It can be either of acute origin or can be of chronic nature.

ETIOLOGY:
1. Vesico ureteric Reflux is the commonest cause.
2. Inadequately treated acute Pyelonephritis.
3. Renal Tuberculosis.
4. Metabolic Disorders like - Diabetes, gout.
5. Urinary obstruction - due to stones, stricture, B.H.P.
6. Neurogenic bladder - Tabes Dorsalis, paraplegia.

CLINICAL FEATURES:
1. Constitutional Symptoms: Features of vague ill health, lassitude, malaise and low grade fever are seen.
2. Pain: in the loins which is dull and aching is constantly present.
3. Urinary Disturbances: in the form of increased frequency and dysuria are generally seen.

4. Hypertension is frequently present particularly in Secondary pyelonephritis.
5. Pyrexia: Attacks of fever exceeding 37.8°c are seen frequently.
6. Anaemia: of normochromic and Normocytic type is seen.

DIAGNOSIS:
1. By complete History and case Taking.
2. Urine Examination: shows Protein uria, casts and micro-organisms.
3. Intravenous Urography: will show the reduced size of Kidneys with localised contraction of renal substance associated with clubbing of the associated calyces.
4. Urine Culture.
5. Micturating Cystourethrogram (MCU) is helpful in diagnosing VUR.

MANAGEMENT:
1. Any underlying abnormality of urinary tract should be corrected.
2. The full course of antibiotics are given for at least 7 days.
3. Fluid Intake: Patients are advised to increase the total fluid intake to 2-3 litres/day.
4. To practise frequent micturition, to keep the bladder empty.
5. Surgical correction by Nephrectomy is done in case of unilateral PyeloNephritis.

Q-3. Describe Acute Nephritis in children with it's management.
(1974 w.Bengal, 1974 Supp, 1975 Supp, 1977, 1983, 1988, 1991 Supp, 1992.)

Ans. Acute Glomerulo Nephritis is one of the commonest renal disease of infective origin seen in children.

ETIOLOGY:
1. It is usually due to streptococal infections. Therefore it is called PRIMARY ACUTE NEPHRITIS.
2. It can be seen secondary to :

Excretory System

a. Membranoproliferative disease of Kidney.
b. SLE.
c. Serum Sickness.

CLINICAL FEATURES:
1. MODE OF ONSET: It can be either with oedema or puffiness of face or with urinary disturbances or with marked constitutional symptoms.
2. OEDEMA: It usually affects the face with bagginess of lower lids. The puffiness with facial pallor gives rise to a NEPHRITIC FACIES.
3. HYPERTENSION: The elevation of B.P ocurs in majority of cases. It usually persists for a week then gradually subsides.

If it remains uncontrolled it may lead to Hypertensive encephalopathy leading to confusion, headache, vomiting epileptic fits etc.

4. IMPAIRED RENAL FUNCTION: oliguria with acute Renal failure may develop in very late stage.

MANAGEMENT:
1. COMPLETE REST: The patient is advised to have complete bed rest which reduces the risk of pulmonary oedema and Hypertensive crisis.
2. RESTRICTION OF FLUIDS: The intake of fluids should be restricted.
3. DIET: Low protein diet. If patient has persistent oedema then dietary sodium should also be reduced.
4. HOMOEOPATHIC MANAGEMENT: Uva ursi, Helleborus and Viola Tricolor can used, if indicated by totality.
5. HOMOEOPATHIC MANAGEMENT: Uva ursi. Hellebo-

Q-4. A patient who is male aged 70 yrs comes to you with B.H.P. What are likely to be his main Symptoms? How would you treat him (1987.)

Ans. The patient with prostatic enlargement will present with following symptoms:
1. FREQUENCY: It is the earliest symptom. At first it is nocturnal and the patient is obliged to get up to micturate twice or thrice at night.

Gradually the frequency becomes progressive and is present both during the day as well as night.

2. URGENCY: The patient cannot wait for the urine. As soon as he feels the urge he must go, otherwise, it will spoil the underclothing.
3. NOCTURIA: He passes more water at Night.
4. DIFFICULTY IN MICTURITION: He must wait patiently for the urine to start. It decreases on straining.
5. STREAM: is usually poor and variable, it stops and starts again then dribbles.
6. PAIN: It may be complained of either with cystitis or retention of urine.
7. HAEMATURIA: Ocasionally the patient will present with passing of drops of blood in urine.

TREATMENT:

1. SABAL SERRULATA: It is one of the excellent remedies for prostatic enlargement. It is usually associated with epididymitis and urinary difficulties in the form of obstructed flow or even enuresis.

There is complete Sexual Neurasthenia. The organs usually feel cold to touch.

2. FERRUM PICRICUM: There is pain along the entire urethra. Smarting at the neck of bladder and penis. Frequent micturition at night with full feeling and pressure in rectum.

It may be associated with Hypertensive epistaxis.

3. CHIMA PHILLA: It is indicated in Senile Hypertrophy when CYSTITIS IS VERY WELL MARKED.

There is constant urge to urinate with passage of turbid, offensive and ropy urine. There is a sensation of ball in the perineum.

The patient must strain before the flow comes. He can urinate only by standing with feet wide apart and body inclined forward.

Q-5. What are the Symptoms of Acute Urinary Tract Infection? How would you treat such a patient with Homoeopathic drugs? (1976, 1977, 1979.)

Ans. SYMPTOMS OF ACUTE U.T.I. :
1. ONSET: is usually sudden with onset of fever, chills and rigors.
2. CONSTITUTIONAL SYMPTOMS: There are severe malaise, bodyaches, pallor, nausea and vomiting.
3. PAIN: There is dull aching at times, severe pain in the loins.
   The loins are tender on palpation.
4. URINARY DISTURBANCES: There is increased frequency of urination with painful micturition. There is passage of blood in urine.

The patient cannot stand the site of urine, it is very offensive.

TREATMENT:
1. CANTHARIS: It is one of the excellent remedies for acute as well as chronic U.T.I. There is constant and frequent desire to pass urine.

   There is scalding pain in urethra as well as fullness in the region of bladder while passing water.

   The pains are usually worse immediately after drinking water.

   Water and coffee are completely intolerable for the patient. The urine is loaded with cells, casts and often the Red cells.

   It is generally associated with catarrh of gastro intestinal tract where jelly like mucus is passed in stools.
2. CHIMAPHILLA: See Q-4.
3. CANNABIS SATIVA: It is a good remedy for U.T.I. when it is of gonorrhoeal origin. There is extreme, scalding pain in the urethra while urinating. The urethra is so painful that he cannot walk properly, must walk with legs apart.

   The stream is generally split with painful urge.
4. APIS MELLIFICA: It is a good remedy for U.T.I. when the last drop passed burns and smarts. There is burning and soreness when urinating. Urine is loaded with lots of pus and mucus. There is bag like swelling of lower eyelids.

Q-6. What are the causes of Renal Calculus? Suggest 4 Homoepathic drugs with their top most symptoms. (1987 Supp.)

Ans. The following are the causes of calculus formation in the Kidneys:
1. RENAL INFECTION: The infection by streptococci, urea spliting organisms are responsible.
2. DIETETIC: The deficiency of vit A causes desquamation of epithelium which acts as a factor for calculus.
3. ALTERED URINARY SOLUTES AND COLLOIDS: Usually the weather changes effect the conc of urine thereby altering the ratio.
4. PROLONGED IMMOBILISATION: From any cause can be responsible.
5. HYPERPARATHYROIDISM:
6. INADEQUATE URINARY DRAINAGE: When ever there is obstruction to the flow it will favour the calculi formation.

HOMOEOPATHIC DRUGS:
1. BERBERIS VULGARIS: It is one of the known remedies for calculus specially in the persons of gouty and Rheumatic diathesis.

There is burning pain in the region of one or both the loins, with bubbling sensation.

The pains are constantly shifting from one place to another. There is marked burning while passing water. Urine is thick passed with mucus and mealy sediment.

There is pain in the thighs and loins on urinating. Frequent urination with burning in urethra when not urinating.

The complaints are worse by motion and on standing.
2. SARSAPARILLA: It is also an excellent remedy for renal calculus when the pains are very severe and cause depression.

There is colic and backache at the same time. There is severe pain at the conclusion of urination. Urine dribbles while sitting.

Urine is scanty, slimy and bloody with sediments. It is especially useful in (R) sided calculus when the pains travel

from the Kidney in a downward direction.
The complaints are worse at night, after urinating.
3. LYCOPODIUM: It usually corresponds to Carbon-itrogenoid constitution of grauvole's who suffer constantly from gastric and urinary disturbances.

There is constant pain in back before urination and is relieved after flow is established.

The urinary stream is slow and broken, must strain. There is polyuria at night.

The urine is heavily loaded with red sediment.

It is generally associated with flatulence and sour eructations.

The complaints are worse on (R) side, from heat and from 4-8 P.M but better by motion.

4. TEREBINTH: It is helpful in calculus when Haematuria is persistent. There is intense burning in the region of Kidneys with drawing pains extending down to the hip.

There is strangury with bloody urine. Urine has a strong odour of violets, is scanty and suppressed. Constant tenesmus of bladder is seen.

Q-7. What are the causes of bloody urine. Give the management with Homoeopathic drugs.
(1982, 1975 Supp, 1977.)

Ans. **CAUSES:**
1. CONGENITAL ABNORMALITIES: Polycystic Kidneys, Horse shoe Kidneys, mobile Kidneys.
2. INFECTIONS: Pyelonephritis; T.B. of Kidney, Glomerulo nephritis.
3. TRAUMATIC: Ruptured Kidneys.
4. TUMOURS: Hypernephroma, CA of bladder.
5. VASCULAR CAUSES: Renal infarction, sickle cell anaemia, malignant hypertension.
6. BLEEDING DIATHESIS: Seen in Sickle cell traits, Haemolytic anaemias, Leukaemia.
7. DRUGS AND CHEMICALS: Use of aspirin, antibiotics.
8. MISCELLANEOUS: Exercise induced, Loin pain and Haematuria Syndrome.

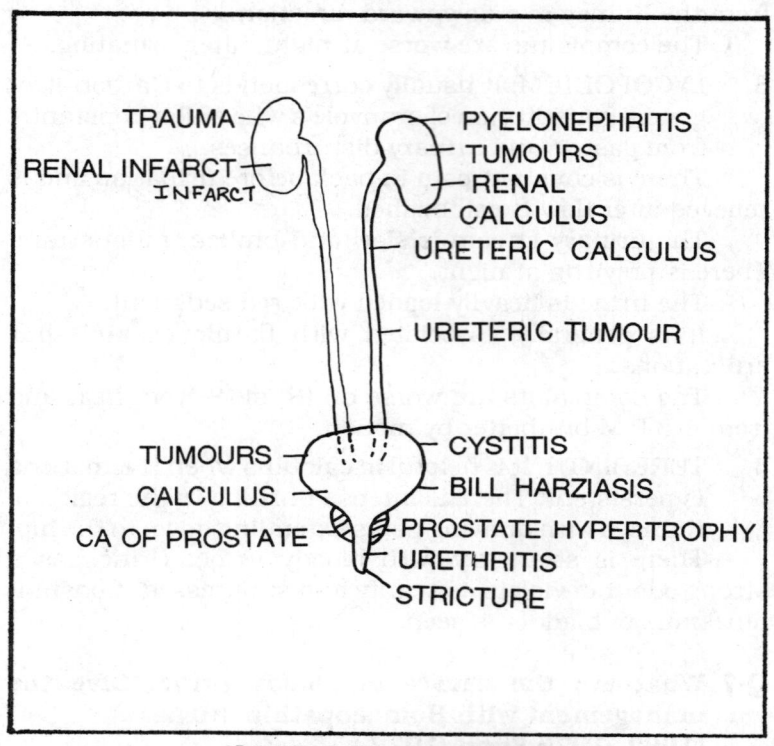

(CAUSES OF HAEMATURIA)

MANAGEMENT:
1. Reassurance to the patient.
2. To assess the general condition by noting pulse, B.P, R.R. and general look.
3. If the general condition is O.K. wait and watch, if not keep the patient ready for general treatment of shock. If needed blood transfusions can be given
4. To correct and remove any underlying cause.

HOMOEOPATHIC MANAGEMENT
1. TEREBINTH: See Q-6.
2. CROTALUS HORRIDUS: It is a remedy suited to the persons of bleeding diathesis.

The urine is dark and bloody with presence of casts. It is generally albuminous, dark and scanty. It acts more particulary on the (R) Kidney. The complaints are worse on (R) side, in open air and from jar.

3. MERC COR: It is also an efficient remedy for Haematuria when there is constant tenesmus of bladder with frequent passage of bloody urine. There is intense burning in urethra.

Urine is scanty, hot and burning with bloody greenish discharge. It contains lots of albumen. There is strong perspiration after urinating.

All the complaints are worse at night and better by rest.

4. THLASPI BURSA: It is an anti Haemorrhagic and anti uric acid remedy.

There is frequent desire to urinate. Urine is heavy, phosphatic. It is good for chronic cystitis with dysuria and spasmodic retention.

The urine contains brick dust sediment urine often comes in little jets.

5. MILLEFOLIUM: It is one of best Remedies for any kind of Haemorrhages from the orifices. There is usually painless bleeding and the blood is generally bright red in colour.

Q-8. A patient lying un--conscious with convulsions and uraemic odour, pupils contracted, not reacting to light; marked vomiting no thirst. How will you manage such a case. (1985)

Ans. MANAGEMENT OF COMA

1. POSITION IN BED: The patient should be nursed with the head in a flat position. He should be kept in semiprone position in order to avoid falling back of tongue.

Frequent change over of the position is necessary to prevent lung congestion.

2. ENSURE PROPER RESPIRATION:
a. keep the tongue forward.
b. oxygen inhalation.
c. Use of Respiratory stimulants.

3. ENSURE PROPER CIRCULATION
a. Parenteral fluids like glucose (isoline can be given.)
b. Use of vaso despressor drugs in case of shock.
4. CARE OF BOWEL AND BLADDER:
a. Catheterisation
b. Saline or soap enema.
5. CARE OF SKIN:
a. Frequent change of position in bed.
b. Care of oral cavity to prevent fungal infections.
c. Alcohol or spirit rub with powdering of skin.
6. CARE AND CONTROL OF SECONDARY INFECTIONS: with antibiotics.

SPECIFIC TREATMENT:
1. TREATMENT OF HYPERKALEMIA: I.V calcium gluconate 10-20 ml in 50% Solution of glucose should be given.
2. DIALYSIS: It is the only method of reviving the patient along with good general care.

Q-9. Give the causes of Renal failure with clinical features and Homoeopathic management. (1983)

Ans. See Q-12. for chronic Nephrosis.

Q-10. Describe signs, Symptoms and management of chronic Interestitial Nephritis. Give the Homoeopathic Remedies. (1983 Supp.)

Ans. See Q-2.
For Homoeopathic management See Q-6.

Q-11. Describe the causes and clinical features of chronic Nephrosis. Discuss the role of diet and Homoeopathic drugs. (1985)

Ans. **CHRONIC NEPHROSIS:** is a special type of Parenchymatous nephritis. It is characterised by the lipoid degeneration of Kidney tubules without any inflammatory signs. Clinically it shows marked oedema, albuminuria, hyperchloesteraemia and hypothyroidism.

Excretory System

ETIOLOGY:
It is always secondary to lesions of kidney.
1. INFECTIONS: Chronic Pyelonephritis, Renal T.B.
2. HYPERTENSION: malignant and non malignant.
3. DESTRUCTIVE LESIONS OF KIDNEY: Glomerulonephritis, Polyarteritis Nodosa, SLE etc.
4. OBSTRUCTION IN URINARY TRACT: Due to Bilateral calculus, prostatic enlargement.

CLINICAL FEATURES:
It usually occurs in the following 3 stages.
1. Stage of diminished Renal Reserve
2. Stage of Renal Insufficiency.
3. Final stage of Renal Failure.

The symptoms can be discussed according to the various systems involved.

SYSTEM	SYMPTOMS	SIGNS
RENAL	Nocturia. Increased Thirst	Proteinuria. Abnormal Urinary Sediments.
CARDIOVASCULAR	Breathlessness Orthopnoea Chest pain Oedema	Fatigue Hypertension. Pericarditis. Circulatory over load. Depletion of Blood volume
G.I.T	Anorexia. Nausea. vomiting. Hiccough. Diarrhoea.	Foetor. ulceration of oral cavity. Parotitis.
NEURO MUSCULAR	Cramps. Weakness. Drowsiness. Fits. Hallucinations. Stupor progressing to coma.	Asterixis. Loss of sense of Vibration and light, touch.

HAEMATO-LOGICAL	Bruises. Epistaxis. Dyspnoea Fatigue	Anaemia. Bruises.
SKIN	Itching.	Skin is dry. Pigmentation. Scratch marks.
SKELETAL	Bone pains.	Rickets in children.
OCULAR	Sore eyes. Falling vision.	Congested eyes. Detachment of Retina. Corneal calcification.

MANAGEMENT:

1. DIET:
a. Low protein diet with 50-55 kcal/kg body weight per day.
b. Restrict the intake of potassium.
c. Sodium intake should be restricted.
2. TREATMENT OF HYPERKALEMIA: Give I.V calcium gluconate in 50% solution of glucose.
3. SALT AND WATER INTAKE: It should be restricted according to the condition of the patient.
4. USE OF DIURETICS: Diuretics like Frusamide or lassix can be used.
5. CORRECTION OF ANAEMIA: The only thing to prevent haemolysis and maintain the Haemopoetic balance is to keep blood urea level below 30 m mol/litre by diet or by dialysis.
6. RENAL OSTEO DYSTROPHY: Secondary Hyper parathy roidism and osteo malacia can be controlled by reduction of serum Phosphate by diet or by supplementation with calcium Carbonate 1-3 gm/day.
7. HYPERTENSION: Specific therapy for the control of Hypertension is given.
8. DIALYSIS: It is usually a last resort in the medical practise to keep the metabolic disorder in some balance and to keep the patient surviving.

HOMOEOPATHIC DRUGS
1. BERBERIS VULGARIS: See Q-6.
2. UREA: It is not a well proved remedy but is clinically indicated in Renal dropsy with albuminuria. Features of uraemia are very well seen. The urine is thin and of low specific gravity. It is given in low dilutions.
3. TEREBINTHA: See Q-6

Q-12. How to differentiate Haematuria from Haemoglobin ura? what are the causes of Haematuria? How do you manage it. (1982)

Ans. Take the urine sample centrifuge and allow it to cool down. Now perform the confirmation test for the presence of R.B.C by the following test:
1. BENZIDINE TEST: Dissolve a pinch of benzidine in glacial acetic acid. Add 2ml of previously boiled and cooled urine to 1 ml of clear benzidine solution and mix.

Add 1ml of fresh 3% $H_2 O_2$ (Hydrogen peroxide). A green or blue colour within 5 minutes is confirmatory for the presence of Red cells.

2. Take the centrifuged urine. Put a drop of it over a glass slide. Now examine it under the microscope. The presence of R.B.C is confirmed.

The presence of Haemoglobin can be confirmed by SPECTROPHOTO METRIC ANALYSIS.
For second part see Q-7.

Q-13. Discuss the management of a case of Uraemia mentioning 2 Homoeopathic medicines (1976.)
Ans. See Q-11.

Q-14. What is Blood Pressure ? What are the conditions that control B.P ? Discuss the clinical features and complications with treatment of Renal Hypertension. (1978 supp, 1992)

Ans. BLOOD PRESSURE : It can be defined as the lateral pressure exerted by the blood column while flowing in the vessel wall. It has 2 components Systolic and Diastolic.

CONDITIONS THAT CONTROL BLOOD PRESSURE:

The B.P is dependent on many factors which in turn control also. They are

1. CARDIAC OUTPUT: It is directly related to the cardiac output More is the output of ventricle per minute more will be the blood pressure recorded.
2. PERIPHERAL RESISTANCE: It is the resistance felt in peripheral arterioles when the blood column flows. It is inversely proportionate to the blood pressure. More is the peripheral resistance less will be the Blood pressure.
3. CONDITION OF ARTERIAL WALL: The blood pressure is dependent on the arierial wall and its conditions. In arteriosclerosis the peripheral resistance is decreased thereby the blood pressure is increased.
4. BLOOD VOLUME: The B.P is directly related to the blood volume, more is the volume of blood in the flowing column, more is the Blood pressure.

CLINICAL FEATURES:

Usually the Renal Hyper tension has varying presentations.

1. ASYMPTOMATIC: with vague presentations of body aches and general weakness.
2. OEDEMA: It may present as facial puffiness on the lower lids, which on investigation shows the underlying Renal Hypertension.
3. PROTEINURIA: It may present with proteinuria when 2-3 gm/day are lost in the urine. It will further add to the puffiness.
4. HAEMATURIA: microscopic or macroscopic haematuria may occur.
5. URAEMIA AND RENAL FAILURE: It is the grave presentation of Renal Hypertension when there is dryness of mouth with difficult breathing. All the features of end Stage Renal failure are present.

COMPLICATIONS:

1. Renal failure and Uraemia.

Excretory System

2. Haemorrhages
3. Malignant Hypertension
4. Hypertensive encephalopathy
5. Chronic Nephrosis
6. Death.

MANAGEMENT:
1. Correction of any underlying cause.
2. Diet: See under Nephrotic Syndrome
3. General management as for uraemia.
4. Drugs like Rauwalfia, Belladona, Glonoine, etc. can be used.

Q-15. What is Nephrotic Syndrome? Describe the clinical features and History with management.
(1981, 1982, 1989, 1991 Supp.)

Ans. Nephrotic Syndrome is a triad of Oedema, protenuria and Hypoproteinaema irrespective of the etiology.

CLINICAL FEATURES:
1. AGE AND SEX: It is more common in children of 2-3 yrs of age with predominence in males.
2. OEDEMA: It is usually peripheral involving the limbs specially the lower limbs.

   It may also be seen on face, abdomen and sometimes on the whole body.

   Intense oedema of scrotum or vulva may also occur. It will lead to ANASARCA.
3. GASTRO INTESTINAL SYMPTOMS: Anorexia with nausea and vomiting and severe malnutrition.
4. BLOOD PRESSURE: There may be varying periods of hypertension leading to permanent changes with the development of Chronic Nephritis.
5. GENERAL SYMPTOMS: Features of tiredness, leathargy muscle wasting, infections, dyspnoea may occur.

MANAGEMENT:
1. DIET: Usually a high protein diet with low sodium in take should be given.
2. USE OF DIURETICS: Diuretics are useful but should be used with caution if the patient is very oedomatous and Hypovalemic.

3. USE OF ANTIBIOTICS: Prophylactic dose should be given to prevent the development of peritonitis and septicaema.

Q-16. A patient aged 30 yrs is brought to you with generalised oedema. What is your miasmatic understanding? How do you manage? Give the indications of Apis, Apocyanum, Digitalis and china. (1984, 1991 Supp.)

Ans. The patient with the oedema of renal origin usually goes in the favour of PSORO SYPHILITIC BACKGROUND.

According to the theory of chronic diseases, Psora is a fundamental cause that prevails behind every disease. The etiology of the renal diseases always leads to the PROGRESSIVE DESTRUCTION OF RENAL PARENCHYMA.

For management See Q-15 and 11.
1. APIS: See Q-5.
2. APOCYANUM: It is very good remedy for dropsy of renal and cardiac origin where there is excessive vomiting. With this the respiration is short and unatisfactory; constantly Sighing. A DIMINISHED FREQUENCY OF URINE WITH LOW PULSE IS A GOOD INDICATION FOR APOCYANUM.
3. DIGITALIS PUERPURA: There is continous urging in drops. Urine is dark, hot and burning with sharp cutting or throbbing pain at the neck of bladder.

There is a constant sensation as if a straw was being thrust back and forth.

It is usually troublesome at night.

With this there is marked dyspnoea and frequent desire to take a deep breath.

The pulse is usually slow, intermits at 3rd, 5th and 7th beats.

The patient feels worse when sitting errect and is better when empty stomach and in open air.
4. CINCHONA: It is a good remedy for dropsy resulting from loss of vital fluids and exhausting discharges.

The skin is extremely sensitive to touch but hard pressure relieves. It is associated with coldness and cold sweat all over the body.

Excretory System

There is noctural diarrhoea which is generally painless with marked prostration.

There is a marked tendency for haemorrhages of bright red colour from any and every orifices of the body.

Q-17. Write short notes on:
1. Haematuria (1978, 1983, 1983 Supp, 1988.)
2. Haemoglobin uria (1988)
3. Hyper Nephroma (1988 Supp)
4. Hydronephrosis (1988 Supp)
5. Blood urea levels. (1987)
6. Cystitis and its management (1987)
7. Creatinine clearance (1989)
8. Renal Hypertension (1991)
9. Urinary Casts (1991, 1992)
10. 3 glass Test for Haematuria. (1992)
11. uraemia: (1974 Supp.)

1. **HAEMATURIA: (See Q-7)**
2. **HAEMOGLOBINURIA:** The presence of Haemoglobin in the urine is called Hburia.

CAUSES:
1. Blackwater fever.
2. Extensive burns.
3. Paroxysmal Haemoglobinuria.
4. Poisoning by mushroons, Potassium Chlorate.
5. Haemolytic Anaemias.

DIAGNOSIS: is established by Spectrophotometric analysis of urine where it should be differentiated from Haematuria.

The presence of HB in urine gives a Smoky COLOUR.

3. **HYPERNEPHROMA:** It is the commonest neoplasm of the Kidneys.

It is an Adenocarcinoma. It usually arises in the cortex from the preexisting adenoma.

PATHOLOGY: It is a tumour of spherical shape, moderate in size. It usually arises from the upper pole of the Kidney. It is yellow to dull white in colour.

MICROSCOPICALLY: It shows the presence of alveoli of cubical or cuboidal cells.

CLINICAL FEATURES:
1. It is more commonly seen in adult males.
2. Intermittent Haematuria.
3. Pain in the loins may be present.
4. A rapidly developing varicocele should always be an INDICATION FOR HYPERNEPHROMA

SPREAD BY: 1. Blood stream into renal veins
2. Lymphatics: to the lymph nodes of hilar area of Kidneys.

TREATMENT:
1. Nephrectomy with Radiotherapy

4. **HYDRONEPHROSIS:** It can be defined as the ASEPTIC DILATATION of renal calyces either partially or in total due to obstruction in the outflow of urine.

ETIOLOGY:
FOR UNILATERAL:
1. Presence of aberrant vessels which over lie the ureters.
2. Idiopathic Retroperitoneal filbrosis.
3. CA of prostate, cervix.
4. Inflammatory stricture of ureter.

BILATERAL:
1. Congenital stricture of urethral meatus.
2. CA of bladder involving both the ureters.
3. Inflammatory or Traumatic urethral stricture.

PATHOLOGY: The calyces are usually dilated and the parenchyma of Kidneys is destroyed by pressure atrophy.

CLINICAL FEATURES:
1. Females are more commonly affected than males.
2. Dull constant pain in the region of loins.
3. Ocasionally attacks of RENAL COLLC may occur.
4. Haematuria may also occur.

DIAGNOSIS: By Intravenous urography

5. **BLOOD UREA LEVELS:** Blood urea is a product of metabolism and breakdown of body proteins taken in the diet.

Excretory System

Normally the levels are between 15-40 mg/100ml.

Any alteration in the Kidney function will cause a rise in Blood urea levels.

The blood urea levels rise only when the GFR is approximately halved.

DISADVANTAGE: The urea production varies with protein intake or increased catabolism of body protein.

There fore it cannot be taken as an accurate judge of the Kidney functions.

6. **CYSTITIS AND ITS MANAGEMENT**

The inflammation of urinary bladder and its mucosa by organisms of varying etiology is called CYSTITIS.

ETIOLOGY:
1. Inadequate or incomplete emptying of bladder.
2. The presence of calculus, foreign body or neoplasm.
3. Lowered general resistance from recurrent diseases.
4. More commonly seen in females.

CLINICAL FEATURES:
1. FREQUENCY: of urination both during the day and night is well marked.
2. PAIN: It varies from mild to moderate. It is felt suprapubically. The pain is referred to the tip of penis.
3. HAEMATURIA: The passage of a few drops of blood stained urine is noticed.
4. PYURIA: The presence of pus cells is simply diagnostic.

MANAGEMENT:
1. To remove any predisposing or precipitating cause.
2. Take plenty of fluids.
3. Frequent bladder emptying should be practised.
4. Use of Antibiotics.

7. **CREATININE CLEARANCE:** One of the diagnostic of Renal function tests is the creatinine clearance.

It should be measured if calculation of GFR from S. creatinine is likely to be erroneous due either to wasting, obesity, oedema or pregnancy.

It is best performed on two consecutive 24 hr urine collections and single blood sample between them.

The (N) endogenous value for males is 97-140 ml/minute. In females it is 85-125 ml/minute.

It is much more an ACCURATE WAY OF MEASURING G.F.R.

8. **RENAL HYPERTENSION:** See Q-14.
9. **URINARY CASTS:** They are the products of coagulation of albuminous material in the lumen of renal tubules. They have following features in general.
1. They are not found in the urine of specific gravity less than 1010.
2. They get dissolved quickly in the alkaline urine.
3. They are usually formed in the distal and collecting tubules.
4. They have parallel sides, broken ends, no internal structure and have various shapes.

They can be of various types:
1. HYALINE CASTS: They are pale, colurless, Homogenous, transparent and cylindrical in shape. They are soluble in water.
2. GRANULAR CASTS: When hyaline casts contain granules they are termed granules. The granules are from degenerating epithelial cells.
3. WAXY CASTS: They usually have a dull grey or colourless way appearance. They are larger than Hyaline casts.
4. FATTY CASTS: They are usually the bulk of fat droplets deposited on the surface of granular or Hyaline casts.
5. CELLULAR CASTS: they can be
a. Red cell casts.
b. Leucocytic casts.
c. Epithelial casts.

IMPORTANCE:
1. They are usually found in acute and chronic Glomerulonephritis, Pyelo nephritis and degenerative diseases of Kidney.

10. **3 GLASS TEST FOR HAEMATURIA:**
It is one of the classical tests for knowing the level of lesion in the urinary tract. For this 3 clean glass tubes or beakers are taken.

The patient is asked to pass the urine and kept in 3 beaker or jars.

Consequently the urine forms 3 layers in each of them. The blood from the urethra which is in the Ist jar forms the first layer.

The blood from bladder which is generally split and changed in colour, often clotted. Comes from the bladder.

The blood which comes from the Kidneys is generally thoroughly mixed.

11. **URAEMIA:** See Q-11.

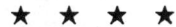

6. ENDOCRINE SYSTEM

Q-1. Discuss acromeagly; it's clinical features and findings on examination. Name important drugs. (1987 Supp, 1988.)

Ans. Acromeagly is a disease of adult life characterised by growth in bulk of the bones of extremites due to Hyperactivity of the pitutiary gland.

CLINICAL FEATURES:
1. SKELETAL CHANGES: There is enlargement of hands and feet. They are spade like. Enlargement of facial bones with LANTERN LIKE JAW (PROGNATHISM) The clavicles are thickened and the teeth are widely spaced.
2. SOFT TISSUE CHANGES: Tongue is enlarged with difficulty in articulation. Nose and lips become thickened. Skin becomes greasy and hyperpigmented. Mammary glands also slow hyperplasia.
3. CARDIOVASCULAR CHANGES: Hypertension, Cardiac failure may be seen.
4. RESPIRATORY CHANGES: Hoarseness of voice with a change in tone of it.
5. METABOLIC CHANGES: Diabetes mellitus develops in few cases.
6. GENERAL FEATURES: like Headache and vomiting usually develop
7. DUE TO PRESSURE UPON ADJACENT OPTIC CHIASMA: AND ADJACENT NERVES: Initially there is bitemporal Hemianopia later blindness develop.

FINDINGS ON EXAMINATION:
1. Spine shows Kyphosis or scoliosis.
2. SKIN: shows hyperpigmentation multiple neurofibroma and papillomatous growths.
3. EYES: Bitemporal Hemianopia, palsies of III, IV and VI

Endocrine System

cranial nerves.
4. THYROID is enlarged.
5. TONGUE: Shows macroglossia.
6. X-RAY: Shows tufting of the terminal phalanges broadening of the epiphysis of long bones. with increased air sinuses of the skull.
7. In females: galactorrhoea and in males gynaecomastia is seen.

HOMOEOPATHIC DRUGS:
1. Thyroidinum
2. Chrysorabinum.
3. Kali Iod -
4. Phosphorus

Q-2. Describe Tetany in detail. Mention its treatment. (1988 Supp.)

Ans. TETANY: Can be defined as a condition developing due to absolute or relative deficiency of Parathyroid Hormone secretions.

It is characterised by an increased excitablity of peripheral nerves.

CAUSES:
It can be either due to decreased Serum Calcium or due to alkalosis.

HYPOCALCAEMIA	ALKALOSIS
1. Malabsorption	Repeated vomitings
2. Chronic Renal failure	Excessive intake of oral alkalis.
3. Acute Pancreatitis	Hyperventillation.
4. Osteomalacia	
5. Hypoparathyroidism	

CLINICAL FEATURES:
IN CHILDREN:
1. A characteristic triad of carpopedal Spasm, stridor and convulsions are seen.
2. MAIN D' ACCOUCHEUR'S POSTURE: In this metacarpo phalangeal joints are flexed. I.P. joints of fingers

and thumb are extended, with thumb in a position of opposition.

IN ADULTS:
1. MENTAL SYMPTOMS: They usually vary from minor disturbances to major Psychoses.
2. SKIN AND NAIL CHANGES.
a. Nails become brittle and ridged.
b. Permanent teeth show the evidence of Hypoplasia
c. Fissures at the angle of mouth.
d. Numbness and tingling around the mouth.

SIGNS:
1. CHOVSTEK'S SIGN: Contraction of facial muscles by tapping over the facial nerve in the front of lobe of ear.
2. ERB'S SIGN: The muscles show increased excitability to galvanic stimulation.
3. TROUSSEAU'S SIGN: Carpopedal spasm can be reproduced by compressing the arm with the sphygmomanometer cuff and maintaining systolic pressure for 1-5 minutes.

TREATMENT:
1. In acute cases give calcium gluconate intravenously
2. LOW PHOSPHORUS: diet should be given. Milk, milk products, fresh fruits, nuts should be reduced.

Q-3. Mention the causes of glycosuria. Discuss briefly the complications and treatment of Diabetes mellitus: (1978 Dms, 1988 Supp.)

Ans. **GLYCOSURIA:** The presence of glucose in the urine is called glycosuria. The following can be seen as the various causes of glycosuria.
1. Diabetes mellitus.
2. Renal glycosuria.
3. Pregnancy glycosuria.
4. Emotional: due to excessive mental strain, trauma or excitement.
5. Raised Intra cranial pressure.
6. Infections and Toxemias
7. Severe Exertion.

COMPLICATIONS OF DIABETES MELLITUS:

1. **DIABETIC RETINOPATHY:** It is one of commonest cause of blindness in adults between 30 and 65 yrs of age. It is characterised by the following changes:
   1. MICROANEURYSM: They appear as minutely discrete, Circular dark spots near to but separate from the Retinal vessels.
   2. HAEMORRHAGES: They usually occur in the deep layers of retina. They are usually blot Haemorrhages.
   3. HARD EXUDATES: They are characteristic of diabetic retinopathy. They usually result from the leakage of plasma from abnormal retinal capillaries
   4. SOFT EXUDATES: They are called cotton wool spots seen on opthalmoscopic examination.
   5. NEOVASCULARISATION: They usually arise from mature vessels on the optic disc or the Retina.
   6. VENOUS CHANGES: They include venous dilatation beading and increased tortusity of veins.
2. **DIABETIC NEUROPATHY:** It can be discussed under the Autonomic Neuropathy and Somatic Neuropathy.

A. SOMATIC: It can be under the following types
1. Symmetrical Sensory Polyneuropathy.
2. Asymmetrical motor Diabetic Neuropathy.
3. Mono Neuropathy.

B. AUTONOMIC NEUROPATHY
1. PUPILLARY: Pupil size is decreased. There is delayed or absent response to light.
3. CARDIOVASCULAR: Postural Hypotension.
- Resting Tachycardia.
- Fixed Heart Rate.
Sudden Cardiac arrest.
4. GASTRO INTESTINAL TRACT:
- Dysphagia
- Abdominal fullness with nausea, vomiting and Nocturnal diarrhoea.
5. VASOMOTOR
- Feet feel cold constantly.
- Dependent oedema.
- Bullae formation

6. GENITOURINARY
- Difficulty in micturition with in continence of urine,
- Recurrent urinary Tract Infections.
- Impotency
7. SUDOMOTOR
- Gustatory Sweating
- Nocturnal Sweats
- Anhidrosis fissures in feet
8. DIABETIC FOOT: It can be either primarily neuropathic or completely ischaemic in origin.

PRIMARILY NEUROPATHIC	ISCHAEMIC
- warm.	cold.
- Bounding Pulses.	Absent pulses.
- Diminished Sensation.	Sensations intact.
- Pink skin.	Skin blanches on elevation.
- Anhidrosis.	
- Callous formation.	
- Cracks and Fissures.	
- Painless ulceration.	Painful ulcers.
- Digital gangrene.	
- Charcot's joints.	
- Wasting of Interosseous muscles.	
- Clawed Toes.	
- Neuropathic oedema.	Oedema associated with cardiac decompensation.

9. DIABETIC NEPHROPATHY: It usually presents with Renal Failure.
10. NECROBIOSIS LIPODICA DIABETICORUM: is one of the complications of m. membranes.

TREATMENT:
1. DIETARY MANAGEMENT:
a. All carbohydrates should be taken in the form of starches and complex sugars. The intake should vary from 100-250 gm/day.
b. Proteins: Usually 60-110 gm/day

Endocrine System

    c.   Fats: Total intake should be reduced and if possible it should be taken in the unsaturated form.
    d.   Complete abstinence from Alcohol.
    e.   Diabetic foods are to be avoided.
    f.   Diabetic sweetners can be used.
2.   USE OF HYPOGLYCAEMIC DRUGS:
3.   INSULIN: INDICATIONS
    a.   young patients with severe diabetes.
    b.   All children
    c.   Patients who are underweight
    d.   In acute onset of diabetes.
4.   HOMOEOPATHIC MANAGEMENT: The following drugs can be used.
    a.   Syzgium Jambolanum.
    b.   Natrum Phos.
    c.   Acid Phos.
    d.   Cephalandra Indica
    e.   Arsenic Album.

Q-4. How would you differentiate a case of Diabetic coma from Hypoglycaemic coma? Mention the clinical tests you would use to establish the diagnosis. Mention 2 Homoeopathic drugs (1981, 1987.)

Ans. They can be defined as the ACUTE COMPLICATIONS of diabetes which can be differentiated from each other clinically.

DIABETIC COMA	HYPOGLYCAEMIC COMA
1. HISTORY: Too little or no insulin, an infection digestive upsets.	No food, too much insulin, or unaccoustomed exercises.
2. ONSET: Ill health for several days.	In good previous health, related to last injection of Insulin.
3. SYMPTOMS: of glycosuria with dehydration, abdominal pain and vomiting.	Features of Hypogly caemia like sinking sensation in stomach, weakness, hunger, diplopia, lassitude somnolance.

DIABETIC COMA	HYPOGLYCAEMIC COMA
4. a. SIGNS: Dry skin and tongue.	They are moist.
b. Pulse is weak.	It is full and bounding
c. B.P is usually low.	It is (N) or slightly raised
d. RESPIRATION: Air hunger	Shallow or normal breathing
e. REFLEXES: They are diminished.	They are brisk.
5. URINE: Will show the presence of glucose and ketone bodies.	No presence of glucose or Ketone bodies if bladder is recently emptied.
6. BLOOD: shows Hyperglycaemia and Reduced Bicarbonates of plasma.	Hypoglycaemia with (N) Bicarbonates.

CLINICAL TESTS:
1. URINE ANALYSIS: It will show the presence of Ketones and sugars in the sample if it is due to DIABETIC KETOSIS.
2. BLOOD ANALYSIS: Will find presence of sugar and reduced levels of plasma bicarbonates in Ketotic origin.

HOMOEOPATHIC DRUGS:
1. PHOSPHORIC ACID: It is specially suited to those persons who are overtaxed both physically as well as mentally. It owes it's origin in sexual excesses, from seminal losses or from excess of grief or any kind of vital fluid loss.

    The patient is apathetic and indifferent with listlessness and constant desire to sleep.

    The urine is frequent and profuse, loaded with phosphates.
2. OPIUM: It is a very good remedy when there is general sluggishness with complete lack of vital reaction. The patient gives a dull stupid look with complete loss of consciousness.

    There is deep snoring with STERTOROUS BREATH-

ING. There is warm sweat all over the body. It is associated with ABSOLUTE CONSTIPATION. The patient is extremely sensitive to slightest touch, noise and even to pressure.

Q-5. What are the causes and clinical features of Addison's Disease? Mention 4 Homoeopathic Remedies (1977, 1982, 1985, 1991 Supp.)

Ans. ADDISON'S DISEASE: It can be defined as a clinical condition resulting either from absolute or relative deficiency of adrenocortical secretions.

CAUSES:
I. PRIMARY
1. Congenital or acquired enzyme defects
2. Bilateral adrenalectomy 3. Infection of glands.

II. SECONDARY
1. Hypothalmic or pitutiary disease.
2. Glucocorticoid therapy.
3. T.B of adrenals
4. metastasis.

CLINICAL FEATURES:
1. ONSET: is gradual.
2. AGE AND SEX: It is commonly seen in females of 30-50 yrs of age.
3. WEAKNESS AND WASTING: The patient gives a vague complaint of not feeling well. There is progressive asthenia and wasting.
4. PIGMENTATION: It is one of the most important features of Addisons Disease. It is usually seen in skin folds, pressure points like axillae, back of neck, forearm, dorsum of hands.

It is also seen in the mucous membranes in the form of brown to black pigmentary areas.

5. HYPOTENSION: The B.P is usually below 100 mm Hg systolic
6. GASTRO INTESTINAL SYMPTOMS: There is loss of appetite specially a disliking for fatty foods.

The bowels are usually constipated.
7. MISCELLANEOUS FEATURES:
a. THORN'S SIGN: Stiffness of ear cartilage, with scanty axillary and public Hairs.

HOMOEOPATHIC MANAGEMENT:

1. ADRENALIN: It is specially suited to the persons where the SYMPATHETIC SYSTEM is very active.

   There is general slowing of pulse with frequent apoplectic attacks.

   There is frequently a sensation of constriction of throat with anguish.

   Constant abdominal pain with nausea and vomiting.

2. CALC ARSENICUM: It is suited to those persons who are very sensitive emotionally.

   There is palpitation from slightest exertion or from any emotional opsets.

   There is frequent rush of blood to the head before the attack.

3. PHOSPHORUS: It is specially suited to the persons who are lean, thin with narrow chest and fair complexioned with a T.B diathesis.

   The patient complains of empty gone feeling in stomach with constant desire for icy cold things.

   There is great weakness with intense restlessness. There is great drowsiness with frequent spells of waking and short naps.

   There is constant restlessness both physically and mentally.

4. ARSENIC ALBUM: It is a good remedy when there is usually a H/O ptomaine poisoning or poisoning with animal tissues. There is great weakness with prostration but he still moves from one place to another.

   There is usually a low vitality with marked periodicity of attacks.

   The skin is dry, rough and scaly specially during winter months.

   All the complaints are worse at midnight from 12-2 A.M/P.M.

Q-6. What is Diabetes mellitus? Give the signs and symptoms with principles of treatment. (1976, 1984)

Ans. DIABETES MELLITUS: It can be defined as a syndrome resulting from absolute or relative deficiency of pancreatic secretions characterised clinically by the triad of polydipsia, polyphagia and polyuria.

SYMPTOMS:
1. GENERAL SYMPTOMS: of tiredness lethargy, weakness are commonly seen.
2. URINARY SYMPTOMS
a. Increased flow of urine.
b. Nocturia
c. Nocturnal enuresis.
3. GASTRO INTESTINAL:
a. Excessive appetite.
b. Increased thirst.
c. Nausea and vomiting.
4. Weight Loss.
5. PRURITUS: of genitalia manifested inthe form of vulvo vaginitis and Balanitis.
6. Impotency.

SIGNS
1. Weight loss.
2. Urine Examination: showing the presence of glucose
3. Blood Sugar is diagnostic.
4. Gradually diminishing VISUAL ACQUITY.
5. VAGINAL EXAMINATION: shows the presence of white discharge with SCAR MARKS.
6. NEUROLOGICAL: In the initial stages loss of vibration and fine touch.

FOR PRINCIPLES OF R_x SEE Q-3.

Q-7. What are the causes of Polyuria? Give in detail the management of Diabetes mellitus.(1975, 1982 Supp.)

Ans. POLYURIA:
I. PHYSIOLOGICAL
1. Excessive intake of water.
2. Use of Diuretics.
3. Psychogenic Polydipsia.
4. Stimulants like alcohol, tea, coffee
5. High protein diet.
6. Post anuric diuresis.

II PATHOLOGICAL
1. ENDOCRINE DISORDERS
a. D.M.
b. Diabetes Insipidus.
2. RENAL DISORDERS
a. Polycystic Kidneys.
b. Nephrotic Syndrome.
c. Chronic Renal Failure.
3. TOXIC CAUSES
a. Drugs.
b. Lithium Toxicity.

For Part II See Q-3.

Q-8. Discuss the investigations of Juvenile Diabetes mellitus presenting with Acute coma. (1989.)
Ans. See Q-4.

Q-9. Give in detail the Complications of Diabetes mellitus (1979.)
Ans. See Q-3.

Q-10. What is Thyrotoxicosis? Describe the causes, clinical features with 4 Homoeopathic drugs How will you differentiate a thyroid swelling from other swellings in the neck?
(1976, 1978 Supp, 1986, 1989.)
Ans. **THYROTOXICOSIS:** It is a clinical condition resulting from the circulation of excess of thyroid Hormones. It usually indicates an increased activity of the thyroid gland.

It is also called Grave's Disease,/Basedow's Disease.

ETIOLOGY:
1. AGE: It is seen exclusively in the 3rd to 4th decade of life.
2. SEX: It is more common in males.
3. PREVIOUS FORMATION OF NODULAR GOITRE: is etiological specially in secondary cases.
4. HEREDITARY: Genetic factors play an important role.
5. AUTO IMMUNE DISORDER: It is predominantly a disease of auto immune origin.

Endocrine System

CLINICAL FEATURES:
1. GOITRE: An enlarged thyroid gland is called goitre. The largest goitre occurs in young males. There is increased blood flow which is manifested by the presence of thrill or Bruit on auscultation.
2. OPHTHALMOPATHY: The symptoms usually develop due to exposure keratitis. They are
    a. Excessive Lacrymation.
    b. Pain in the eyes.
    c. Loss of visual acquity from corneal oedema or optic nerve compression.
3. PRETIBIAL MYXOEDEMA: It is an infilter ative dermopathy which takes the form of raised pink coloured or purplish plaques on the anterior aspect of the leg which usually extends to the dorsum of the Foot.

    It may give the appearance of PEAU'D ORANGE with the growth of COARSE HAIRS.
4. Flushing of face with capillary pulsations all over the body.
5. The skin is warm and moist to touch.

ORBITAL SIGNS ON EXAMINATION
1. JOFFROY'S SIGN: Absence of wrinkles on forehead on asking the patient look up from the down turn position of eyes.
2. MOEBIUS SIGN: Difficulty in convergence when the object is brought near the eyes.
3. VON GRAFE'S SIGN: Persistent lagging of eyelid below the corneoscleral limbus is a positive sign.

HOMOEOPATHIC MANAGEMENT:
1. IODUM: It is a good remedy for the people who are ill nourished, physically weak with dark complexion, rigid muscle fibres having a T.B diathesis.

    There is ravenous hunger with loss of flesh simultaneously. There is frequent weakness specially when using the stairs.

    There are hot flushes with marked palpitations all over the body. It is associated with undeveloped mammary glands in females.

2. THYROIDINUM : It produces anaemia, emaciation, sweating, headache, muscular weakness with tremors and trembling of the hands and face.

Heart rate is increased with exopthalmos and dilated pupils.

In females it may be associated with uterine fibroid or tumours of breast.

It should be given in High potency.

3. CALC IOD: It is one of the best remedies when the persons of Scrofulous habits are affected specially with enlarged tonsils and glands all over the body.

The thyroid enlargements are seen at the time of puberty.

It is associated with Indolent ulcers accompanying varicose veins.

4. GLONOINE: It is a good remedy when reflex symptoms are experienced maximum in the region of head. There is rush of blood to head with violent pulsations and throbbing of head. The pain is very severe, darting, worse from slightest motion, from least jar and from suppressed menses.

The neck feels full with a constant choking feeling.

HOW TO DIFFERENTIATE

1. A Thyroid swelling always moves on deglutition or when the patient is asked to swallow.
2. It is usually central in position.
3. On palpation Isthmus can be felt in between the 2 lobes of Thyroid.

Q-11. What is obesity? Describe the different factors responsible for it. Plan a diet for such a case. Mention 3 Homoeopathic medicines with their indications for it's treatment. (1983, 1992)

Ans. OBESITY: It can be defined as an excess of adipose tissue. The exact criteria is usually controversial. But an increase in 10% of the total body weight in confirmation with Ideal body weight is considered to be the obesity.

It is one of the commonest disorders in medical practise.

FACTORS

1. AGE: In some people, as the age increases the body weight also increases.
2. SEX: It is more common in females.
3. SOCIO ECONOMIC FACTORS: Those persons who belong to a rich society and background, due to irregular eating habits are more affected.
4. EATING HABITS: Those persons who feed constantly on carbohydrates, eat frequently or take irregularly with constant munching through out the day.
5. GENETIC FACTORS: usually if there is a strong genetic background it also comes as one of the important factors.
6. BEHAVIOUR: If a person is of the anxious personality then he or she eats more and thereby gains weight.
7. ENDOCRINE FACTORS: like Frohlichs Syndrome or puberty adiposity are responsible.
8. LACK OF EXERCISE: and physical activity also add to it.

DIETARY PLANNING:

MEALS	MENU
1. Morning	One cup tea or coffee with Tsp sugar + milk.
2. Break fast	Skimmed milk = 1 Cup 1 Toast Sweet lime
3. LUNCH	mixed vegetable = 1 katori Thin Dal = ½ cup. mixed vegetable salad = ½ plate cooked pumpkin = 1 katori Chapatis: = 2 1 Fruit
4. Evening Tea	Tea 1 cup with 2 Biscuits.
5. Dinner	1 cup Tomato Soup 1 Katori = Curd Thin Dal = 3/4 cup Chapatis = 2

TOTAL CALORIES: If sedentary Habits = 800-1800 cal/day

HOMOEOPATHIC MANAGEMENT

1. **CALC CARB:** It is specially suited to persons of fat, flabby and fair diathesis.

   The female constantly puts on weight with constipated bowels and feels better when constipated. There is excessive sweating which smells sour and suffers from belching and eructations constantly. All the complaints are worse in cold and damp weather.

2. **IODUM:** See Q-10.

3. **FUCUS:** When obesity is associated with Non toxic goitre it is well selected and suited.

   The digestion is slow and passage of flatulence is diminished.

   Obstinate constipation with a feeling as if the head has been compressed by an iron ring.

   It is usually given in mother Tincture.

Q-12. Give the clinical features of cretinism. How will you investigate it. Give 3 Homoeopathic medicines. (1979, 1992)

Ans. INVESTIGATIONS:

1. Serum T_4 with T_3 uptakes: are below normal
2. Serum TSH: is usually raised about 20 mu/litre
3. Serum Cholesterol is markedly elevated.
4. E.C.G: shows low voltage complexes with inverted T waves.
5. Neurological Investigations:
a. Tendon Reflexes are prolonged
b. Nerve conduction velocity is also prolonged.
6. THYROID ANTIBODIES: They are generally present

For other parts Refer to PEDIATRICS Q-4.

Q-13. Give an account of Exopthalmic goitre with 4 drugs (1975 Supp.)

Ans. See Q-10.

Q-14. What are the causes, manifestations, complications of CUSHING'S SYNDROME? Give 4 Homoeopathic Drugs. (1985, 1992.)

Endocrine System

Ans. CUSHING'S SYNDROME: is defined as the symptoms and signs associated with prolonged, inappropriate elevation of free corticosteroid levels.

CAUSES:
1. Primary adreno cortical disease with glucocorticoid excess due to Adenoma or CA
2. Secondary:
a. From pitutiary.
b. Ectopic Acth production
c. Bronchogenic CA.

CLINICAL FEATURES:
1. FACE: is moon shaped with a dusky pale look.
2. ADIPOSITY: In the face, neck and abdomen, less in extremities. It is called BUFFALO TYPE OF OBESITY.
3. Purple striae on abdomen, thighs, breast etc.
4. VIRILISM IN FEMALES: i.e. Scanty or absent menses with growth of hairs on face, upper lip and trunk.
5. Hypertension.
6. Psychological upsets.
7. Less likelihood of allergy.
8. Osteoporosis of bones with Kyphosis.
9. Easy tendency for bruises and striae.

COMPLICATIONS:
1. Hypertensive Heart Disease
2. Diseases associated with Hyper chloesteraemia.
3. Psychiatric: May commit suicide or may become maniacal.
4. Diabetes mellitus
5. Hypokalemia
6. Increased tendency for infections.

HOMOEOPATHIC MANAGEMENT
1. CALC CARB: See Q-11
2. IODUM: See Q-10.
3. FUCUS: See Q-11
4. GRAPHITES: It is suited to females who are fat with costive habits and tendency for delayed menstruation.

There is frequent rush of blood to head and ears with marked congestion.

There is easy sweating which smells like honey. The skin is usually unhealthy where slightest injury causes suppuration.

All complaints are better by riding in the carriage.

The patient is extremely chilly with all the aggravation in cold and damp weather.

Q-15. Give the Differential Diagnosis of Goitre. (1981, 1991.)
Ans.

1.	Simple Goitre	Diffuse Hyperplastic. Nodular goitre.
2.	Neoplastic Goitre	Benign and Malignant.
3.	Toxic Goitre	Diffuse Toxic goitre. Toxic Nodular goitre. Toxic Nodule.
4.	Inflammatory swellings	Dequervan's Disease. Auto Immune Thyroiditis. Riedle's Thyroiditis.
5.	Rare forms	Acute Bacterial Thyroiditis. T.B. Thyroid Amyloid goitre.

Q-16. What is myxoedema? Describe its signs and Symptoms, with investigations and homoeopathic treatment. (1975 Supp 1982.)
Ans. MYXOEDEMA is a conditon due to absolute or relative deficiency of circulating thyroid Hormones.

SYMPTOMS	SIGNS
A. GENERAL	
1. Tiredness, Somnolence.	Goitre
2. Weight gain.	
3. Hoarseness	
B. CARDIO RESPIRATORY	
1. Pain in chest	Bradycardia. Hypertension with H.H.D. Xanthelesma.

Endocrine System

SYMPTOMS	SIGNS
	Pericardial and pleural effusion.
C NEURO MUSCULAR	
1. Aches and pains.	Delayed relaxation of tendon
2. muscle stiffness.	reflexes.
3. Deafness.	carpal Tunnel Syndrome.
4. Depression, psychosis.	Cerebellar ataxia.
	myotonia.
D. HAEMATOLOGICAL	
1. weakness.	macrocytosis.
	Anaemia - Iron deficiency
	- Pernicious
	Or - Normochromic
E. SKIN	
a. Itching.	Skin is dry, flaky.
	Alopecia.
	Vitiligo.
F REPRODUCTIVE	
1. Menorrhagia.	Infertility.
2. Galactorrhoea.	
G G.I.T.	
1. Constipation.	Ascites.
	Ileus.

INVESTIGATIONS:
1. Serum T_3 and T_4 are low
2. TSH is increased.
3. Low Serum Sodium .
4. Choesterol levels are raised.

HOMOEOPATHIC MANAGEMENT
1. CALC CARB - See Q-11
2. GRAPHITES - See Q-14
3. THYROIDINUM - See Q-10
4. IODUM: - See Q-10

Q-17 Enumerate the causes of Burning Feet Syndrome. Give the etiology, pathology, clinical features with complications and management of Diabetic Foot. (1992.)

Ans. **CAUSES**
1. ENDOCRINE
1. Diabetes Mellitus
2. Hyperthyroidism
3. Cushing's Syndrome
2. ALCOHLISM
3. DRUGS AND TOXINS
1. Carbon Tetra Chloride and its derivatives
2. Certain Heavy metals like Arsenic, Platinum
4. INFECTIVE NEURITIS
1. Gullan Barie Syndrome
2. Landry's paralysis
5. PSYCHOGENIC
Seen usually in old females and obese patients.
6. DEFICIENCY DISEASES
1. Vit B12 Deficiency
2. Pellagra
3. Vit E deficiency.

For 2nd part See Q-3.

Q-18. Write Short Notes on:
1. **Hyper Cholesteraemia (1987, 1988 Supp, 1992)**
2. **Cretinism (1983, 1991, 1982, 1992)**
3. **Diabetic Neuropathy (1991)**
4. **Signs of Hypothyroidsm (1991 Supp)**
5. **Retinal Lesions in Diabetes (1991 Supp)**
6. **Myxoedema (1978)**
7. **Ketosis (1975 Supp)**
8. **Acromeagly (1979)**
9. **Cushing's Syndrome (1979, 1981)**
10. **K.W Syndrome (1979, 1982 Supp)**
1. **HPERCHLOESTERAEMIA:** It is one of the common metabolic disorders in which there is increased levels of circulating lipids.
   It can be placed in two categories:
1. PRIMARY:
2. SECONDARY
It can manifest itself in the following ways:
1. Ischaemic Heart disease

Endocrine System

2. Cerebrovascular Accidents.
3. obesity.
4. Xanthe lesma or Xanthomas.
5. Clinical findings show an increase in the Total fatty acids, Triglycerides and lipids. The Normal value is 150-250 mg./100 ml.

MANAGEMENT:
1. DIET: Low energy, low fat diet should be taken. Increased proportion of unsaturated fats should be included in the diet.
2. Complete abstinence from alcohol.
3. Use of lipid lowering drugs.
4. In Homoeopathy drugs like crategus, Adrenaline and Iris Tenax have a questionable value in controlling the Hyperlipidemia.

2. **CRETINISM** - Refer to Q-4 of Pediatrics
3. **DIABETIC NEUROPATHY** See Q-3.
4. **SIGNS OF HYPOTHYROIDISM** - See Q-16.
5. **RETINAL LESIONS IN DIABETES** - See Q-3
6. **MYXOEDEMA** - See Q-16.
7. **KETOSIS:** The diabetic Ketoacidosis is a medical emergency which should be treated in the Hospital.

PRECIPITATING FACTORS:
1. Too little or no insulin.
2. Infections.
3. Gastric upsets.

MANAGEMENT:
1. The administration of I.V fluid or normal saline to correct dehydration.
2. Potassium Replacement.
3. Administration of antibiotics if infection is present.
4. Administrationof Insulin by I.V route.

8. **ACROMEAGLY:** See Q-1.
9. **CUSHING'S SYNDROME:** See Q-14

10. **K.W SYNDROME:** It is called Kimmelstil wilson Syndrome. The renal disease of diabetic origin is called K.W Syndrome.

It is becoming more common since diabetic patients live much longer than a few decades ago.

It is found equally in mild or in severe cases of diabetes of 10 years or more years standing.

The progressively severe albuminuria and Hypertension result in uraemia, Cardiac Infarction or a cerebro vascular catastrophy. It is generally associated with a chronic urinary infection.

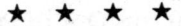

7. PSYCHIATRY

Q-1. Mention the features of Acute Depression. How would you treat this condition? (1987, 1988.)

Ans. The clinical features can be discussed under
1. PSYCHIC SYMPTOMS: There is depression of mood. It usually varies from individual to individual.

The patient is most distressful in the early morning on waking up or at the end of the day. There is complete loss of pleasure in life, loss of interest in self and others.

Low self esteem, self blame and Hopelessness are predominent.

The patient often has suicidal thoughts. Severe depression is accompanied by feelings of guilt and worthlessness which are usually delusional in nature.

2. SOMATIC SYMPTOMS
a. Sleep Disturbances - Initial insominia, early morning waking or Hyper somnia.
b. Fatigue.
c. Headache.
d. Vague pains all over the body.
e. Anorexia.
f. Weight change.
g. Constipation.
h. Reduced Sexual desire.
i. Poor concentration.
j. Psychomotor Retardation.

TREATMENT:
1. Psychotherapy.
2. Use of Antidepressive drugs.
3. Use of Electro convulsive therapy.
4. Homoeopathic drugs like Aurum met, Platina, Nux

moschata and Zincum can be used.

Q-2. Describe various types of Schizophrenia. Mention the general treatment. (1988 Supp.)

Ans. Schizophrenia is a group of mental illnesses characterized by specific psychological symptoms leading to a disorganisation of the personality

VARIOUS TYPES:

1. SIMPLE: It usually occurs in males in the age of 15-20 yrs. It usually affects the disturbances, Social unresponsiveness, thinking disturbances, behaviour disturbances with delusions and Hallicinations are present.

PROGNOSIS: is not good.

2. HEBEPHRENIC: It starts with an acute onset at the age of 20-30 yrs.

    Thinking disturbances are most marked.

    There is regression, childish behaviour, inappropriate affect, silliness with hallucinations are present.

3. CATATONIC: It starts with an insidious onset and affects equally both the sexes.

    Symptoms of catatonia are most marked.

    Autism with features of disturbed behaviour are present.

4. PARANOID: Delusions of suspiciousness are characteristic. Disorganisation of speech and thoughts with hallucinations are seen. Personality is usually preserved with a good PROGNOSIS.

TREATMENT:

1. Psycho therapy.
2. Electro convulsive therapy.
3. Occupations or work therapy is the best way to treat these patients.

Q-3. Give the Indications of Ignatia, Lachesis, Nat mur and Nux moschata in Hysteria. (1982.)

Ans. IGNATIA: It is suited to those females who are emotionally very sensitive.

There is changeable mood with silent Brooding. Patient is sad, tearful and melancholic.

The complaints usually develop after a shock or grief or any disappointment in life.

There is constant sighing, and sobbing with a weeping tendency when alone. The patient does not communicate. All the complaints are full of CONTRADICTIONS.

All complaints are made worse by tobacco and by consolation.

2. LACHESIS: It is suited to the personalities of melencholic disposition. The patient is sad, and amiative specially in the morning.

These is no desire to mix with the world. There is great loquacity with constant changing over of the topics.

The patient has immense jealousy and is full of suspicion. She is restless and uneasy, does not wish to attend the business wants to be off somewhere all the time.

She is full of religious insanity but with great fear and dreams of snake.

There is derangement of time sense.

All the complaints are worse at the change of life, from pressure.

3. NATRUM MUR: It is a remedy which usually antidotes the ill effects of grief, fright anger etc. It is suited to the patients of depressed, melancholic tendencies.

There is great depression with a weeping tendency. She weeps when alone but is always worse by consolation.

The patient is extremely irritable and gets into a passion about trifles.

She is awkward and hasty drops things from hands.

4. NUX MOSCHATA: It is suited to those females who have a tendency for FAINTING FITS.

There is marked changeability of the mood with alternate laughing and crying. She is very forgetful and always confused.

Q-4. Describe various types of depression with clinical features and complications. Mention the general treatment. (1992.)

Ans. Clinically depression can be classified into

I. TYPICAL DEPRESSION   II. ATYPICAL DEPRESSION

Typical can again be discussed under:
1. Autogenous   2. Neurotic or Reactive Depression
a. Psychotic Depressive Reaction.
b. Involutional Depression.
c. Depressive phase of maniac depressive psychosis.

1. PSYCHOTIC DEPRESSIVE REACTION: It starts between the age of 25-30 yrs. It is more commonly seen in women than men.

The classical features of depression like sadness of mood, poverty of ideas, psychomotor retardation, early morning insomnia, constipation, dryness of mouth, anorexia, diurnal variction of mood.

The attack usually lasts from 6 months to 18 months.

2. INVOLUTIONAL DEPRESSION: It occurs for the first time around the period of involution i.e. around the age of 45-55 yrs.

In females it is related to menopause. Besides the characteristic features of depression, these patients usually suffer from anxiety, hypochondriasis and PARANOID IDEATION.

3. MANIAC DEPRESSIVE PSYCHOSIS: It is characterised by alternating cycles of maniac psychosis and depressive psychosis.

They usually suffer from the fluctuating moods between elation and depression.

A family History of the other members suffering from the same illness is significant.

II NEUROTIC OR REACTIVE DEPRESSION: It occurs usually in persons of anxious, melancholic or obsessive personality. The patient shows all the symptoms of depression except those of Autonomic Nervous system dysfunction.

ATYPICAL DEPRESSIONS: The group refers to the clinical syndrome of depression associated with pneumonia, influenza, malignancy, arteriosclerosis, heart disease, endocrine disturbances etc.

COMPLICATIONS:
1. Suicidal tendencies.
2. Maniacal attacks at times.

TREATMENT:
1. Psychotherapy.
2. Use of Electro convulsive therapy (ECT).
3. Drug Therapy.
4. Occupational and work therapy.

Q-5. What is Neurosis? Describe it's clinical features. How will you treat such a case? (1980.)

Ans. It is the commonest forms of psychoneurosis. The anxiety reactions are frequently displayed in normal adaptation to environmental stress.

CLINICAL FEATURES:
1. Anxiety is the foremost symptom. There is a strong feeling of insecurity and problems are magnified.
2. Fears of bodily or mental illness, of suicide and death are common.
3. Acute panics lasting minutes or hours characterised by paroxysmal terror and emotional distress occur.
4. There is fear of society, to meet people, to walk in the traffic and may sit in the House all day.
5. Sleeplessness contantly from the frequent ideas.
6. Visceral symptoms :
a. G.I.T: Nausea, vomiting, waterbrash, heartburn, diarrhoea, constipation.
b. VISUAL: Blurring of vision.
c. SEXUAL: Seminal emissions.
a. NEUROLOGICAL: Twitchings of mucles.
7. Effort syndrome: It is characterised by breathlessness, giddiness, palpitation, tachycardia, sweating, pain and exhausation.

TREATMENT
1. Reassurance and psychotherapy.
2. To rule out any precipitating factors.
3. To boost up the general morale of the patient.
4. Advice good nutritious balanced diet.

5. Following Homoeopathic drugs can be used.
   a. ARGNITRICUM   b. SELENIUM   c. ALUMINA
   d. GELSEMIUM   E. IODUM.

Q-6. Write short Notes on
1. **Reactive depression and its treatment (1988 1991 supp)**
2. **Maniac depressive syndrome (1988 Supp)**
3. **Schizophrenia (1987)**
4. **Hysterical behaviour (1983, 1985, 1987.)**
5. **Neurasthenia (1985)**
6. **Acute mania (1989)**
7. **ECT (1989)**
8. **Alcohlism (1991.)**

Ans.

1. **REACTIVE DEPRESSION See Q-4**

2. **MANIAC DEPRESSIVE SYNDROME/PSYCHOSIS See Q-4.**

3. **SCHIZOPHERINA See Q-2.**

4. **HYSTERICAL BEHAVOUR**: Hysteria is a type of neurosis characterised by somatic or psychological symptoms without any organic basis.

   This behaviour is usually seen in females of shallow emotional relationship, who constantly dramatize and exhibit seeking attention.

   It is purely psychogenic in origin which cannot be explained on anatomical basis or any organic basis.

   This behaviour is exhibited only in the presence of public. The patient is indifferent to the symptoms even though they are incapacitating.

5. NEURASTHENIA: It is chronic nervous exhausation which is characterised by the fatigue and some degree of anxiety.

CLINICAL FEATURES:
1. Tiredness both physical and mental. It is generally not relieved by a night's rest and is always precipitated by some factors.
2. Emotional instability with irritability and loss of control.

3. Patient becomes egocentric and introspective.
4. Lack of concentration with a peculiar kind of headache a constant dull aching tightness radiating from the frontal region into the back of head.
5. Feeling of wooliness or cloudiness in various parts of the body.
6. Sleeplessness.
7. Menstruation may be irregualr in females.

TREATMENT:
Same as of Neurosis.

6. **ACUTE MANIA :** It is a type of functional psychosis, the symptom triad is characterised by elevation of mood, flight of ideas and increased psychomotor activity.

CLINICAL FEATURES:
1. DISTURBANCE OF MOOD: The patient is very active, jolly, and sparkling with excessive satisfaction with his own self and circumstances
Euphoria is very well marked.
2. DISTURBANCES OF THINKING: Flight of ideas is frequently seen. Stream of ideas is very rapid, goal keeps on changing and he jumps from one subject to another. Talk is forceful and pressure of speech is raised.
3. DISTURBANCES OF BEHAVIOUR: Restlessness and overactivity doing everything in excess. Putting into action many schemes but not completing any. Degradation of conduct with sexual assaults and exposures.
7. **ELECTROCONVULSIVE THERAPY:** It is one of the modes of treatment used in psychatric disorders. It is indicated when the risk of suicide is so great that one cannot wait for the delayed therapeutic effect of antidepressant drugs.

INDICATIONS: 1. Acute mania.
2. Depressive stupor.
3. Psychoneurosis:
In this electrodes are placed on the respective parts of the brain and the current is passed.

8. **ALCOHLISM:** The consumption of alcohol is increas-

ing day by day but males have more alcohol related problems than the females.

CRITERIA FOR ALCOHOL DEPENDENCE:
1. Priority of drinking over other activities.
2. Tolerance of effects of alcohol.
3. Subjective compulsion to drink.
4. Repeated withdrawl symptoms.
5. Relief of withdrawl symptoms by drinking.

PROBLEMS DUE TO ALCOHISM:
1. SOCIAL PROBLEMS: Absentism from work, unemployment, marital tension, child abuse, financial difficulties.
2. PSYCHOLOGICAL PROBLEMS: like depression, morbid jealousy are seen.
3. WITHDRAWL SYMPTOMS: It is seen in the form of tension on waking in the morning with tremors, visual hallucinations, memory disturbances and epilepsy.
4. VITAMIN DEFICIENCIES: usually vit B complex deficiency occurs leading to the development of korsakofs psychosis or wernicke's encephalopathy.
5. TOXIC EFFECTS ON BRAIN: There is period of amnesia with intoxication.

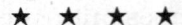

8. GASTROINTESTINAL SYSTEM

Q-1. A 40 yr old male patient presents to you with Ascites mention various etiological factors and give it's management. (1975 Supp, 1977, 1978, 1979, 1982 Supp, 1988, 1991)

Ans. The collection of fluid in the peritoneal cavity is called ASCITES.

ETIOLOGY:
1. Tubercular peritonitis.
2. Neoplasms of the peritoneum.
3. Congestive cardiac failure.
4. Extra as well as Intra Hepatic obstruction of the portal vein by either sepsis, foreign body or secondary metastasis.
5. Hypoalbuminaemia seen in
   a. Malnutrition   b. Nephrosis   c. Protein losing enteropathy.
6. Beri Beri.
7. myxoedema.
8. Epidemic Dropsy.
9. Ovarian Diseases: meig's syndrome; Ascites with pleural effusion and ovarian cyst.

MANAGEMENT:
1. DIET: should be low in sodium and rich in proteins.
2. DIURETICS: They are of immense value.
3. TREATMENT OF THE UNDERLYING CAUSE: like Anti tubecular treatment for T.B, vit B_1 for Beri Beri, Digitalis therapy for cardiac failure.
4. ABDOMINAL PARACENTESIS: It should be done if
   1. There is severe abdominal discomfort.

2. Cardiac or respiratory embarrasment.
3. Anorexia and dyspepsia
4. Patient is refractory to full medical Therapy.
   At a time about 250-300 ml of fluid should be taken out.
5. Homoeopathic drugs like Apocyanum, Convalaria, Adrenalin, Adonis vernalis can be used in physiological doses.

Q-2. Discuss Irritable Bowel Syndrome. How would you differentiate from ulcerative colitis?   (1988.)

Ans. It can be defined as the irritability of colon producing characteristic symptoms such as constipation, diarrhoea, abdominal pain caused by functional abnormalty of bowel activity in the absence of any demonstrable organic disease.

ETIOLOGY:

1. MOTILITY DISORDERS OF INTESTINES: The pattern and sequence of motility show considerable abnormalities.
2. EMOTIONAL FACTORS: Immature, rigid and perfectionist behaviour is more frequently associated. Anxiety neurosis or depression usually worsen the condition.
3. DIETARY ARTICLES: such as acids, fruits, salads and tomatoes may act as luminal spasmogens.
4. Some cases may follow episodes of infective colitis and amoebiasis.

CLINICAL FEATURES:

1. Females are more common sufferers than males.
2. There is painless functional diarrhoea.
3. Painless simple constipation.
4. Alternating diarrhoea and constipation.
5. Bloating of abdomen.
6. Pain due to spasm of colon and small intestine.
7. Vague symptomatology like abnormal bowel habits ranging from constipation to diarrhoea, pellet like stools, increased gastrocolic reflex flatulence relieved by belching, capricious appetite with insomnia.

Gastrointestinal System

CLINICAL EXAMINATION: does not show any abnormality

ULCERATIVE COLITIS	IRRITABLE BOWEL SYNDROME
1. It is an inflammatory condition of unknown etiology characterised clinically by recurrent attacks of bloody diarrhoea.	It comprises an increased motility of the gastro intestinal tract without any organic basis.
2. AGE AND SEX: It is seen between 20-40 yrs of age with equal incidence in both sexes.	It affects the middle aged females more.
3. ETIOLOGY: Idiopathic	As mentioned above
4. GENETICS: has a definite role to play.	No known role. But it may run in families.
5. PATHOLOGY: Diffuse inflammation of colonic mucosa with infilterations.	only hyperaemia of colonic mucosa is seen.
6. CLINICAL FEATURES	
a. ONSET: Sudden, fulminating with a chronic History.	It is always sudden relating to some past significant event.
b. Attacks of bloody stools.	There is increased frequency without any blood.
c. Constitutional Symptoms are very marked.	They are not seen.
7. COURSE: is variable without any actual relief.	The course is prolonged with remissions and exacerbations.
8. COMPLICATIONS: like polyposis, conjuntivitis, arthritis, piles, fistulae are common.	only nutritional deficiencies are seen as complications in later part of disease.
9. STOOL EXAMINATION shows the presence of blood and mucus.	There is steatorrhoea.

10. RADIOLOGICAL DIAGNOSIS a. mucosa is fragile with hyperaemia, bleeds on touch. b. Barium Enema shows reduction in length and calibre of the colon.	No such changes are evident.

Q-3. A 30 yr old patient comes to you with pain in (R) lower abdomen. Mention various causes. How would you investigate a case of Renal colic. (1988 Supp.)

Ans. CAUSES OF PAIN IN RIGHT LOWER ABDOMEN:

1. ACUTE APPENDICITIS: A careful history indicates the initiation of pain first in the periumbilical area which later on shifts to (R) Iliac fossa.
   Pain is associated with fever and vomiting. There is usually a past History of short lasting attacks.
2. ACUTE REGIONAL ILEITIS: In this there is usually a previous long lasting H/O intestinal colic and diarrhoea. A tender mass can be felt inthe right lower abdomen by pelvic examination. The patient when complains of pain in right Iliac fossa with other complications like anal fissure, fistula or oedomatous skin tag then the diagnosis is certain.
3. RENAL COLIC WITH OR WITHOUT URETERIC SPASM:
   There is severe pain in (R) or (L) loin which is usually reffered down to the Lower abdomen. It compels the patient to bend double.
   It is generally associated with difficulty in urination which is often burning in nature Haematuria may or may not be associated but STRANGURY is well seen.
4. T.B OF ILEOCAECAL REGION: There are recurrent attacks of pain with diarrhoea, weight loss and anaemia. The evening rise of temperature is very diagnostic.
5. AMOEBIC TYPHLITIS: Diarrhoea with pain is the main feature. On examination a thick, tender colon can be

Gastrointestinal System

palpated.
6. ACTINOMYCOSIS: of caecum and appendix is associated with pain and lump in (R) Iliac region, multiple sinuses discharging sulphur granules are usually diagnostic.
7. ACUTE SALPINGITIS: In females is the commonest cause of pain in lower abdomen. It usually starts at the time of menstruation or immediately after abortion or delievery
   It is associated with fever and difficulty in micturition.

INVESTIGATIONS:
1. Clinical History Taking.
2. Urine Examination routine and microscopic Will show the presence of pus cells and R.B.C with or without oxalates.
3. Plain X-Ray KUB will show the calculus in the shadowy areas of kidneys.
4. Intravenous urography

Q-4. A 40 yrs old gentle man admitted as Haematemesis and malena. Discuss the Differential diagnosis and general management. (1975, 1975 Supp, 1977, 1981, 1982 Supp, 1988 Supp. 1992.)

Ans. Vomiting of blood is called Haematemesis and blood passed in stools is called malena.

ETIOLOY
I. SWALLOWED BLOOD :
1. Epistaxis.
2. Haemoptysis.
3. Bleeding from mouth and throat.
4. malingering.
II. DISEASES OF OESOPHAGUS :
1. Reflux oerophagitis.
2. Peptic ulcer syndrome.
3. Ruptured oesophageal varices.
III. DISEASES OF STOMACH :
1. Acute and chronic gastritis.
2. CA of stomach.
3. Mallory weiss syndrome.

4. Peptic ulcer syndrome.
IV. PORTAL OBSTRUCTION :
1. Cirrhosis.
2. Portal vein Thrombosis.
V. ACUTE FEBRILE DISEASES:
1. malignant scarlet fever.
2. malignant variola.
3. Subacute Bacterial Endocardits.
VI. BLOOD DISEASES :
1. Purpura.   4. Leukaemia.
2. Scurvy.   5. malarial cachexia.
3. Haemophillia
VII. MISCELLANEOUS
1. Prolonged jaundice
2. Systemic Lupus erythematosus (S.L.E)
3. Malignant Hypertension.

GENERAL MANAGEMENT.

1. ADMISSION TO HOSPITAL: is essential because a small bleed may become life threatening.
2. REST: Complete physical as well as mental rest is essential.
3. SEDATION: is also essential to avoid anxiety and panic
4. OBSERVATION: of Pulse, B.P and general condition of the patient is necessary.
5. IV DRIP (N) Saline should be given intravenously
6. If situation is grave and uncontrollable give blood transfusions
7. Correction of underlying cause.
8. FEEDING: To aid absorption, gastric lavage is first done then intragastric feeds are given to the patient.
9. USE OF DRUGS: to control bleedings.

Q-5. Discuss pancreatitis; its complications and management. Give its Homoeopathic Treatment. (1988 Supp.)

Ans. Inflammation of pancreatic islets due to factors of varying etiology leads to Pancreatitis
Clinically it can be either.
1. ACUTE PANCREATITIS. It can be defined as an acute

condition presenting with abdominal pain associated with raised pancreatic enzymes in blood due to inflammation of pancreas.

ETIOLOGY:
1. Alcohlism.
2. Gall stones.
3. Viral Infilteration of pancreas.
4. Reaction to drugs.
5. As an auto Immune Disease.

CLINICAL FEATURES.
1. It is seen more commonly in males of 40-50 yrs.
2. Onset is sudden and dramatic.
3. PAIN: Severe pain in the epigastric region is felt which is usually referred to the back.
   Pain is associated with nausea and vomiting.
4. Ecchymosis with bluish discolouration of loins and umbilical area is seen.
5. Jaundice may be seen in few patients.

CHRONIC PANCREATITIS: It is defined as a continuing inflammatory disease of pancreas characterised by irreversible morphological changes and typically causing pain with permanent loss of function.

ETIOLOGY:
1. Alcoholism.
2. Pancreatic duct obstruction by stricture/Trauma.
3. Cystic fibrosis.
4. Idiopathic.

CLINICAL FEATURES:
1. Epigastric pain being referred to the back is increased after taking alcohol.
2. Weight loss.
3. Diarrhoea
4. A tender mass is felt in the epigastrium.

COMPLICATIONS:
1. Shock.
2. Pulmonary Insufficiency.
3. Hypercalcemia.
4. Pseudocyst.

5. Infection   6. stricture of colon.

HOMOEOPATHIC TREATMENT:

1. IODUM: It is a good remedy suited to the persons of dark complexion with rigid muscle fibres and coarse hairs.

   There is voracious appetite but he losses flesh while living well. There is pain in the epigastrium which is aggravated when on empty stomach. He becomes anxious if does not eat.

   There is generally a tendency for diarrhoea. The stools are loose and contain undigested food particles.

2. IRIS VERSI COLOR: There is great burning throughout the alimentary canal. There is sour vomiting which is bloody and biliary in nature.

   There is reduced appetite with profuse flow of saliva.

   Flatulent colic with watery stools and burning at anus. All the complaints are worse in evening and at night but better by motion.

3. ABROTANUM: It is also one of the efficient remedies where the patient is very thin, skinny and wrinkled.

   There is tendency for lienteric stools with oozing of moisture from navel.

   There is great emaciation with a Rheumatic Diathesis

Q-6. Describe the varieties, signs and symptoms, clinical features and complications of Abdominal Tuberculosis. Name 4 drugs. (1987 Supp.)

Ans. The T.B of abdomen is very common in India. Following types of T.B abdomen can be found.

1. Peritoneal T.B. - ascitic, loculated and obliterated type.
2. Intestinal T.B.
3. T.B of mesentric lymph nodes.
4. Renal T.B.
5. Suprarenal T.B.
6. Vertebral T.B. or pott's disease.
7. T.B. of uterine adenaxae.
8. T.B. of liver, stomach which is generally very rare.

1. INTESTINAL T.B.

CLINICAL PATTERNS:
1. PRIMARY T.B.: Primary complex may form in the intestine with its 3 components particulary in infants taking unpasteurised milk.
2. POST PRIMARY OR SECONDARY T.B. It is common and may take the following shapes:
1. Milliary T.B.
2. Secondary T.B. enteritis or ulcerative type of Intestinal T.B.
3. Hypertrophic ileocaecal T.B. or primary T.B. enteritis.
2. TUBERCULAR ENTERITIS
1. It is usually found in young females.
2. It occurs in the seondary form as a complication of pulmonary T.B. from swallowing sputum. It is due to human strains of T.B. bacillus.
3. usual seat of affection is Ileocaecal region. It can be either Primary or Secondary.

PRIMARY OR HYPERTROPHIC TYPE:
1. There is pain in (R) Iliac Fossa.
2. Anorexia, nausea, vomiting, diarrhoea, weakness, wasting and evening rise of temperature are more marked.
3. Symptoms of intestinal obstruction are more marked.
4. Visible peristalsis may be seen in step ladder pattern.
5. A palpable mass is felt in the (R) Iliac Fossa.
6. Barium meal shows a filling defect.

SECONDARY TUBERCULAR ENTERITIS: In this type the dose and virulence of the organism are more and the host resistance is less, therefore necrosis, caseation and ulceration of intestines develop usually.
1. Onset is gradual with weakness, emaciation, pyrexia and abdominal pain which is felt diffusely all over the abdomen.
2. Symptoms of Intestinal obstruction: like distension of abdomen, vomiting, constipation and increased bor borygmi are complained of.
3. Diarrhoea.

COMPLICATIONS
1. Intestinal obstruction.
2. Stricture of Intestines.
3. Nutritional Impairment.
4. Malabsorption in later stages.
5. Recurrent infections.

HOMOEOPATHIC DRUGS
1. Iodum.
2. Iris versicolor.
3. Thyroidinum.
4. Phosphorus.

Q-7. Differentiate Gastroenteritis from Cholera. As a health officer what preventive measures would you advice in either of the conditions. Suggest 4 Homoeopathic Drugs. (1987 Supp.)

Ans. GASTRO ENTERITIS	CHOLERA
1. EPIDEMOLOGY. It occurs in a single group of people who shared some common meal.	It occurs in epidemic form.
2. INCUBATION PERIOD: From 1-24 hrs.	From few hrs to 5 days.
3. INFECTIVE: No secondary cases occur.	Secondary cases occur
4. INITIAL SYMPTOMS. Vomiting	Diarrhoea.
5. STOOLS: Frequent with mucus and blood, highly offensive.	copious, rice water like non offensive.
6. TENESMUS: Present.	No.
7. DEHYDRATION AND CRAMPS: Distinctly seen.	Very marked.
8. TEMP: Upto 102° F.	It is subnormal.
9. BLOOD PICTURE: Normal.	Shows leucocytosis.
10. ABDOMINAL TENDERNESS: Yes.	It is absent.

ROLE OF HEALTH OFFICER:
1. Identification and Isolation of the cases.
2. To guide the parents/guardians regarding the Hygenic measures.

Gastrointestinal System

3. To provide safe drinking water facilities.
4. To look after the patients with utmost care.
5. Facilities of vaccination if available should be availed of.

HOMOEOPATHIC DRUGS:

1. VERATRUM ALBUM: The diarrhoea and vomiting start at the same time. The stools are profuse and very offensive. It is associated with cold sweat all over the body but specially on face. There is great desire for cold refreshing and juicy things.

2. CAMPHOR: The attack usually occurs in the epidemic form. The stools are generally very scanty; but debilitating. Although the discharges are very less but they are very exhausting. Clinically it is useful in CHOLERA SICCA. The pulse is soft, irregular and later on becomes imperceptible.

3. CUPRUM METALLICUM: It is a good remedy for cholera when cramps are very marked. They are usually felt in the flexors. It is associated with great weakness, coldness and often cyanosis. The tongue is constantly protruding with trembling.

All complaints are better by taking cold drinks or cold water.

4. ARSENIC ALBUM: It is a good remedy for gastro enteritis when complaints are usually resulting from ingestion of ptomaine food and stale foods.

The stools are scanty with smell and is generally worse after midnight. The complaints are associated with extreme restlessness.

There is marked aversion to food and cannot bear even the sight or smell of food.

Q-8. Describe a case of ulcerative colitis. How will you manage it. Discuss the Differential diagnosis. Give 4 Homoeopathic drugs. (1986, 1991 Supp.)

Ans. DEFINITION: It is an inflammatory disease of unknown origin characterised by recurrent attacks of bloody diarrhoea and pathologically by a diffuse inflammation of the colonic mucosa.

ETIOLOGY:
1. It is commonly seen in females of 20-40 yrs of age.
2. There is a definite genetic background.
3. Psychological factors may influence the course.

CLINICAL FEATURES:
1. Onset is insidious with diarrhoea and simultaneous passage of blood and mucus.
2. Pain in Left lower abdomen which is relieved by defecation associated with tenesmus.
3. Constitutional Symptoms: of malaise, fever, weight loss are very marked.
4. EXTRA INTESTINAL MANIFESTATIONS:
a. Apthous stomatitis ·   b.   Erythema nodosum ·
c. Pyoderma gangrenosa ·   d.   Conjunctivitis.

MANAGEMENT:
1. REST: Complete physical and mental rest is essential ·
2. CORRECTION OF DEHYDRATION: and electrolyte losses by I.V route is required.
3. CORRECTION OF ANAEMIA: by repeated transfusions

DIFFERENTIAL DIAGNOSIS:
1. Ischaemic colitis.
2. Amoebiasis.
3. Proctitis due to Herpes Simplex ·
4. Gastroenteritis.
5. Salmonellosis.

HOMOEOPATHIC DRUGS
1. MERC COR: It is a good remedy for ulcerative colitis when there is tenesmus of rectum and bladder at the same time. The stools are passed with tenesmus which is not relieved even after passing stools.

The stools are very offensive, scanty bloody with mucus. More the blood more is the indication. It is generally associated with an infection of throat.

2. IRIS VERSICOLOR: See Q-5.
3. CANTHARIS: It is also good when the stools contain

Gastrointestinal System

shreddings of mucus membrane. There is great burning while passing urine with stools.

It is associated with great tenesmus and burning while passing water. All the complaints are made worse by drinking water and coffee.

4. NUX VOMICA: It is specially suited to the persons of sedentary habits who are very lethargic with tendency for gastric upsets.

There is frequent ineffectual urge to pass stools with great tenesmus which is partially relieved after passsing stools.

The stools are generally scanty and offensive. There is constant inclination to vomit It is associated with great desire to sleep and reduced activity of the brai.

Q-9. Discuss the etiology, pathology, and clinical features of peptic ulcer Syndrome. Give the indications of 4 Homoeopathic medicines with stress being laid on the Role of diet in the management. (1976, 1978 Supp, 1983, 1984, 1985.)

Ans. **ETIOLOGY:**
1. AGE AND SEX: It is seen in 3rd to 4th decade of life. It is more common in males.
2. GENETIC FACTORS: It often runs in families.
3. SMOKING: Incidence is high in smokers.
4. PERSONALITY: It is seen more in anxious personalities and in people with responsible jobs.
5. ASSOCIATION WITH OTHER DISEASES: In association with R.A, hyperparathyroidism, cirrhosis etc.
6. BLOOD GROUP : Persons with B group and O are more prone to develop it.
7. ENDOCRINE FACTORS: It is seen in association with multiple adenoma Syndrome, Zollinger Ellison Syndrome.
8. DIETETIC FACTORS: Irregular diet, highly spicy food with inadequate mastication are contributory.
9. ROLE OF HYPERCHLORHYDRIA: is definite in the duodenal ulcer.

PATHOLOGY: A chronic gastric ulcer is usually larger

than the duodenal ulcer.

The ulcer varies in size but admits the tip of a finger. The floor is situated in the muscular coats of the stomach and gradually the ulcer occupies the posterior wall.

The base is covered by a thin layer of granulation tissue. The arteries inthe neighbourhood show the evidence of end arteritis obliterans. At the margin epithelial proliferation can be seen.

CLINICAL FEATURES:

1. PERIODICITY: The attacks are usually with a periodicity ranging from few weeks to several months period.
2. PAIN: It is epigastric in location. In gastric ulcer it is always felt after eating while induodenal ulcer it is better by eating.
3. HAEMATEMESIS AND MALENA: It is seen in the ratio of 60:40 in gastric ulcer and 40:60 in duodenal ulcer.
4. APPETITE: is good but in gastric ulcer the patient is afraid to eat. While in the other case the patient eats and becomes plumpy.
5. WEIGHT: The gastric ulcer patient is underweight and the duodenal ulcer patient puts on lots of weight.

ROLE OF DIET:

1. The diet should be light, simple, palatable and soothing.
2. It should include lots of milk, milk products, liquids and less of spices.
3. If good diet is given it, usually reduces the chances of remissions.
4. Gives a general feeling of well being to the patient.
5. It is known to promote the healing and will not allow it to proliferate further.

But the research which is still continuing is at present is doubt ful regarding the last mentioned point.

HOMOEOPATHIC DRUGS:

1. BRYONIA: It is a good remedy for P.U.S when pain is felt about 1-2 hrs after meals. There is a feeling as if a stone is placed in the abdomen. The patient is very hungry and eats all the time. There is increased thirst for large

quantities of water at long intervals. The bowels are usually constipated with passage of dry, hard offensive stools.

The pain in abdomen is better by lying still or by pressure.

2. KALI BICHROMICUM: It is a remedy for round ulcers of stomach which are called PUNCHED OUT ULCERS.

It causes severe pain of syphillitic origin The pains are generally worse 1-2 hrs after the meals.

It is associated with coldness in stomach and vomiting of thin stringy material. The patient has inclination to vomit and feels relieved after vomiting. There is great desire for beer. All the complaints are usually worse at Night.

3. BISMUTH: It is a good remedy for gastric ulcer when pain with vomiting is very well marked.

There is severe pain in the epigastrium which goes to the back. The pain is better by bending backward.

It is associated with great depression, he cannot bear solitude and always wants company.

4. STRYCHNINE: There is severe pain with retching and violent Vomiting. It is associated with griping pain in bowels. There is much Irritability with soreness of Scalp. It is generally associated with rigidity of muscles, twitchings and trembling of single muscles.

The complaints are worse in the morning, by touch but better by lying on the back.

Q-10. Discuss the etiology, clinical features along with differential diagnosis of Inflammatory Bowel Disease. Mention important Homoeopathic drugs.(1991)
Ans. See Q-8.

Q-11. Give the management of bleeding from oesophageal Varices (1992.)
Ans. See Q-3 of Liver and Gall bladder.

Q-12. Enumerate the points of difference between Amoebiac and Bacillary dysenery with treatment. (1974, 1975 W. Bengal, 1977, 1978, Supp, 1983, 1989, 1992.)

AMOEBIAC DYSENTRY	BACILLARY DYSENTRY
1. EPIDEMOLOGY: It is usually endemic.	It is epidemically found in temperate climates.
2. INCUBATION PEROID: Fortnights or months.	one week or less.
3. AGE: Uncommon in children.	Common in children.
4. SYMPTOMS	
a. It is a walking dysentry.	Is a Lying down dysentry.
b. Onset is insidious.	Is usually acute.
c. Frequency of stools is not much.	It is marked.
d. Fever is rare.	It is usual.
e. Toxaemia is slight.	It is moderately present.
f. Adominal pain and tenderness variable located on (R) side	It is severe, localised to (L) side
g. Tenesmus is moderate or absent.	usually severe.
5. COMPLICATIONS and sequale are many	They are few.
6. MACROSCOPIC STOOL EXAMINATION	
a. Bulky	Scanty.
b. offensive Faeces intermingled with dark blood and mucus.	They are non offensive with mucus in jelly, like lumps.
7. MICROSCOPIC	
a. Red cells in clumps with less cellular elements	Very cellular with discrete R.B.C.
b. macrophages are scanty.	They are usually present.
c. Degenerated lymphocytes, active E. Histolytica and charcol Leyden crystals are present.	Polymorphs are present.
8. SIGMOIDOSCOPY: shows raised button	They are serpignous ulcers with inflammed mucosa.

Gastrointestinal System

| like ulcers or oval flask shaped ulcers with normal mucosa in between. | |

FOR HOMOEOPATHIC TREATMENT: See Q-8.

Q-13. Write the etiology, symptoms and signs with differential diagnosis and prognosis of CA stomach. (1978 D.M.S.)

Ans. It is one of the commonest malignancy in adult elderly males.

ETIOLOGY:

Although no definite factor is known but Some can be considered as Risk or premalignant factors:
1. Gastric polypi.
2. Pernicious anaemia.
3. Gastritis.
4. cigarette smoking.
5. Patients with a long standing history of dyspepsia.
6. Gastric ulcer.
7. A genetic background.

CLINICAL FEATURES:

The symptoms usually fall into 2 categories. One with well defined Symptom group and other comes under the vague category.

1. NEW DYSPEPSIA AFTER 40: Persistent indigestion occurs in a patient who has never Previously had stomach trouble.
2. INSIDIOUS ONSET: General tired feeling with weakness, Anaemia, Anorexia and asthenia are very marked.
3. OBSTRUCTIVE TYPE: It presents with dysphagia, pain, fulness, belching and vomiting.
4. LUMP: It can be accidentally discovered in the epigastric area.
5. SILENT: It may present with obstructive jaundice, ascites, phlebothrombosis of leg or as TROISER'S SIGN.

DIFFERENTIAL DIAGNOSIS:
1. Peptic ulcer Syndrome.

2. T.B of abdomen.
3. Mallory weiss Syndrome.
PROGNOSIS: It has a poor prognosis with a survival rate of 5-7 yrs.

Q-14. What do you understand by Bacillary dysentry? Describe the Homoeopathic treatment. (1975 Supp, 1978 Supp, 1979, 1981, 1982.)

Ans. It is one of commonest tropical diseases of bowels caused by the Bacilli of Shigella group as Shigella Shiga, S. Sonnei etc.

For Rest See Q-12.

Q-15. What is Colic? What are its varieties? Discuss the etiology, Signs, Symptoms of one such variety Mention 3 Homoeopathic medicines with their indications. (1974 Supp.)

Ans. Colic: is a term applied to spasmodic paroxysmal pain situated in the abdomen.

They can be of
1. Billiary   2. Renal   3. Intestinal types.

The following features are common
1. The pain is extremely severe, sudden in onset
2. The patient is doubled up with pain, becomes restless or rolls about.
3. There is reflex vomiting with pallor and anxiety of face.
4. The pain may be relieved by pressure.

RENAL COLIC: The pain in the region of one or both kidneys is called Renal Colic.

ETIOLGOGY:
1. Renal stones.
2. Infections: Pyelonephritis, T.B.
3. Tumours:

FEATURES:
1. The onset is sudden with severe pain in the region of loins. It may or may not radiate down along the course of ureters.
2. It is made worse by any jar or motion.

3. It is associated with mild fever, vomiting and dysuria.
4. The urine is bloody with intense burning while micturition
   FOR HOMOEOPATHIC MEDICINES See Q-7 of Excretory system.

Q-16. Compare and contrast
1. Intestinal and colonic diarrhoea (1989)
2. T.B and Cirrhotic ascites (1991.)
3. Haematemesis and Haemoptysis (1977)
4. Exudate and Transudate (1991)
5. Benign and malig nant Gastric ulcer (supp. 91)

1. INTESTINAL DIARRHOEA	COLONIC DIARRHOEA
1. Pain colicky in nature.	It is generally painless or with dull aching pains.
2. The stools are associated with mucus only.	They are passed with mucus as well as blood.
3. Signs of malabsorption are seen frequently.	They are not seen.
4. The stools are small in quantity.	They are bulky.

2. T.B ASCITES	CIRRHOTIC ASCITES
1. AGE: usually young or adolescents.	middle age.
2. AMOUNT OF FLUID: is small or moderate.	It is usually large.
3. LIVER: Not enlarged	May not be palpable. If palpable, is firm with regular edges.
4. FEVER: Present.	Is absent.
5. TENDERNESS is present.	is rare.
6. ASCITIC FLUID: is exudate.	is a transudate.
7. OTHER FEATURES: Primary focus in the lungs may be found.	There is emaciation, dyspepsia with impaired liver function and established collateral circulation.

8. PERITONEO SCOPY: Peritoneum is infilterated with small granulomas.	Nodular surface of liver is present.
3. HAEMATEMESIS 1. Blood is vomitted. 2. Blood is acidic and brown in colour. 3. Blood is not frothy. 4. There is no sputum but it may be mixed with food. 5. Past History of gastritis, duodenal ulcer etc. 6. Stools are black and tary. 7. It has a brief episode. 8. Nausea usually precedes the attack.	**HAEMOPTYSIS** It is coughed up. It is alkaline and bright red in colour. Part of it is frothy. Blood is mixed with sputum. Previous History of cough. respiratory illness. They are normal. Episode lasts for few days. It generally does not occur.
4. EXUDATE 1. Appearance: is turbid. 2. Specific gravity is more than 1015. 3. Proteins are more than 2.5 gm/100 ml. 4. Cells are usually lymphocytes.	**TRANSUDATE** It is clear. It is less than 1015. They are less than 2.5 gm/100 ml. Transudate shows the presence of endothelial cells with Ocasional lymphocytes.
5. BENIGN GASTRIC ULCER 1. AGE: Seen in young patients. 2. DURATION OF SYMPTOMS: varies from weeks to years.	**MALIGNANT GASTRIC ULCER** In older individuals. From weeks to months.

Gastrointestinal System

3. SEX: marked male predominence	slight male preponderance.
4. GASTRIC ACIDITY: may be normal or slightly increased	It is usually normal or can be entirely absent.
5. LOCATION: on lesser curvature.	On the greater curvature of pyloric and prepyloric region.
6. SIZE: Less than 2 cm in diameter.	usually more than 4 cm in diameter.
7. RESPONSE TO MEDICAL TREATMENT: is good.	shows a refractory response to treatment.
8. X-Ray: shows a small punched out niche with involvement of surrounding wall.	It demonstrates defect irregular or heaped up margins with induration of surrounding mucosae.

Q-17. A patient comes to you with pain in the epigastrium. What may be the common causes in such a case? Mention at least 3 diagnostic features in each case. (1976)

Ans. The following can be the causes for pain in epigastrium:

1. ACUTE PANCREATITIS: Pain is sudden which is reffered to the back. It is associated with shock and blueness in the region of umbilicus and loins.

2. MYOCARDIAL INFARCTION: In the manifest form of M.I there is usually a past History of pain in chest. The pain is of constricting type with anxiety, lot of sweating and low B.P and pain is reffered to the shoulder or down to the arms. The cardiac enzymes are usually raised.

3. REFLUX OESOPHAGITIS: The patient usually wakes up from sleep at night and gives the H/O overfeeding the last night. It is associated with reflex vomiting and is relieved by antacids.

4. PEPTIC ULCER SYNDROME: The pain in duodenal ulcer is felt 2-3 hrs after meals and in gastric ulcer immediately after eating. It is relieved by eating in duodenal ulcer and is made worse by eating in gastric ulcer.

It is associated with haematemesis and or malena.
5. CASTOMACH: There is usually a History of vague dyspepsia with lump on palpation. There is haematemesis with loss of weight and CANCER CACHEXIA.
6. ACUTE CHOLECYSTITIS: The pain is felt in the middle of abdomen and is reffered to the (R) shoulder. It is associated with belching and fullness and is triggered after meals.

Q-18. A patient comes to you with the complaint of progressive emaciation. What may be the causes of it. How will you investigate such a case to arrive at its diagnosis? Is it possible to cure such a case with the help of homoeopathic medicines if proper diagnosis cannot be made. (1976.)

Ans.   **CAUSES OF EMACIATION**

Although there are lot many causes but the main causes responsible are:
1. Anorexia Nervosa
2. Tuber culosis
3. Diabetes mellitus
4. Cancer of any organ of the body.

INVESTIGATIONS:
1. Blood: TLC, DLC, Hb, E.S.R, Presence of antibodies, Blood Sugar, Liver function Tests, serum amylase. etc.
2. Urine with routine and microscopic both
3. X-Ray of chest, abdomen, and bones.

PART III: Although clinically it is a difficult case to treat. As, if we know, the diagnosis the way of treatment is also to some extent guided. But if good and positive symptoms can be elicited then it can be a good case to tackle clinically and can also achieve good results.

Q-19. Write short notes on
1. **Occult blood in stool (1982 Supp, 1988 Supp.)**
2. **Pseudocyst of pancreas (1988 Supp)**
3. **Serum Amylase (1985, 1986)**
4. **Koilonychia (1974 Supp, 1984)**
5. **Hiccough (1983)**

Gastrointestinal System 133

6. **Halitosis (1989)**
7. **Gingivitis (1978)**
8. **Anorexia (1978)**
9. **Haematemesis (1978)**
10. **Peptic ulcer (1978)**
11. **Dry cholera (1978)**
12. **Dysphagia (Supp 1978)**
13. **CA stomach (1974)**
14. **Murphy's Sign (1975 Supp, 1977 Supp)**
15. **Cheliosis (1975 Supp.)**
16. **Oesophageal varices (1976, 1977 Supp.)**
17. **Plummer vinsan Syndrome (1972.)**

1. **OCCULT BLOOD IN STOOLS:** Blood in stools may appear in steaks or in quantity when from the rectum or large bowel. If it comes from stomach or small intestines it will undergo partial digestion and gives the appearance of TARRY STOOLS Called malaena.

   In any case it reddens the water in which stool is placed and gives a characteristic SPECTRUM

   Occult blood must always be tested for in cases of suspected oozing from an ulcerated surface.

2. **PSEUDOCYST OF PANCREAS:** The collection of fluid in the lesser sac as a complication of acute pancreatitis is called pseudocyst. It is about the size of melon and is present in the epigastric region in the centre. It does not move with respiration and is fixed.

   It is generally tensed and thereby Fluctuation cannot be elicited.

LOCATION: It can be seen either
1. Between stomach and the transverse colon.
2. Between stomach and liver.
3. Behind or below the T. colon.

   TREATMENT: It gradually disappears simultaneously if does not, it requires surgical correction.

3. **SERUM AMYLASE:** It is one of the widely used diagnostic tests for assessing pancreatic function. It is usually liberated by the pancreas, salivary glands, lactating breasts, liver and bile ducts.

   The Amylase activity is defined in terms of Somoygi's

units.

It usually rises within few hours of pancreatic damage and declines after 48 hrs.

CONDITIONS IN WHICH IT IS RAISED:
1. Acute abdomen.
2. Intestinal obstruction with gangrene.
3. Cholecystitis.
4. Ovarian cysts.
5. Perforated duodenal ulcer.
6. Alcohlics:

NORMAL VALUE: 50-100 Somoygi's units.

4. **KOILONYCHIA:** The spoon shaped appearance of nails resulting from iron deficiency anaemia is called koilonychia.
   It can either be congenital or acquired.
   It is usually associated with atrophy of nails.

5. **HICCOUGH:** It is caused by the spasm of diaphragm which occurs at regular intervals but sometimes occurs at the time of closure of glottic aperture producing a typical sound.

In normal human beings the contraction of diaphragm is synchronous with opening of glottis.

ETIOLOGY:
1. GASTRO INTESTINAL It is due to stimulation of phrenic nerve.
   a. Paralytic ileus.
   b. Constipation.
   c. Intestinal dilatation.
   d. Flatulence.
   e. Intestinal obstruction.
   f. Excess of spicy foods.
   g. Tobacco chewing.
2. PSYCHONEUROTIC
3. DISEASES OF THORACIC VISCERA:
   a. Diaphragmatic pleurisy.
   b. mediastinal tumours.
4. NEUROLOGICAL CAUSES
   a. cerebral tumours.
   b. meningitis
5. TOXIC:
   a. Uraemia.   b. Liver failure.

6. **HALITOSIS:** Bad smell from the mouth is called halitosis.

CAUSES:
1. Lack of oral Hygiene.
2. Excessive smoking or tobacco chewing.
3. Tooth cavities.
4. Acute Tonsillitis.
5. Diptheria.
6. Vincent's infection.
7. Bronchiectasis.

MANAGEMENT:
1. Removal of underlying causes.
2. maintainence of oral Hygiene.

7. **GINGIVITIS:** The inflammation of mucosa lining the gums is called gingivitis.

CAUSES:
1. Thrush.
2. Vincent's infection.
3. Drugs.
4. Scurvy.
5. Dental caries.
6. Over crowding of teeth.
7. Mouth breathing.

CLINICAL TYPES :
It can be of
1. Hypertrophic type   2. Ulcerative type

HOMOEOPATHIC DRUGS: like Kreosote, mercsol, Plantago can be tried.

8. **ANOREXIA:** Loss of appetite is called anorexia. It is not always an indication of stomach disease. But it may be present in many general constitutional disturbances such as T.B, malignancy or any infection.

It's main importance lies in its presence in the early stage of gastric cancer.

In cancer of stomach and chronic gastritis there is sometimes no appetite before a meal or a premature feeling of fullness after a few mouth fulls.

In gastric ulcer there is fear of taking food.

Another peculiar type is Hysterical anorexia which is characterised by
1. Refusal to eat.
2. Pronounced loss of weight.
3. Constipation.
4. Slow pulse.
5. Growth of downy hairs on limbs and face.
6. Cold blue extremities.
7. No organic condition is present.
9. **HAEMATEMESIS: See Q-4.**
10. **PEPTIC ULCER See Q-9**
11. **DRY CHOLERA:** It is also called CHOLERA SICCA. In this there is no vomiting or diarrhoea and the patient dies of collapse before these symptoms can take over.

The autopsy shows the presence of lot of fluid in the intestines.

12. **DYSPHAGIA:** Difficulty in swallowing either solids or liquids is called dysphagia.

CAUSES:
1. IN THE MOUTH: Tonsillitis, quinsy, CA of tongue paralysis of soft palate.
2. IN THE PHARYNX: impaction of foreign body, pharyngitis, pharyngeal diverticulum, Hysterical spasm, enlarged lymph nodes.
3. IN THE OESOPHAGUS: Stricture, spasm, neoplasm or bulbar palsy, retrosternal goitre, Thyroid swelling pressing over it.

13. **CA STOMACH:** See Q-13.
14. D.P. MURPHY'S SIGN: It is clinically one fo the commonest way of eliciting the tenderness in the case of Acute Cholecystitis.

To elicit, one places the right hand just below the (R) costal margin on the lateral border of the (R) Rectus.

Moderate pressure is exerted with the fingers to palpate the fundus of gall bladder. The patient is now asked to take a deep breath in, the gall bladder descends and hurts the examining fingers.

The patient will immediately wince with a catch in the

Gastrointestinal System

breath if the organ is inflammed. It is called MURPHY'S SIGN.

15. **CHELIOSIS:** The inflammation of lips and of the corners of mouth is called cheliosis.

It is characterised by dry, cracked lips which are usually oozing with vesication and crushing.

ETIOLOGY:
1. Bad oral Hygiene.
2. Deficiency of vit B12.
3. Streptococcal Infections
4. As a Hypersensitive Reaction to pigment EOSIN of lipsticks.

16. **OESOPHAGEAL VARICES:** See Q-3 of liver and gall bladder

17. **PLUMMER VINSON SYNDROME:** It is a common clinical condition developing in females due to iron deficiency anaemia. It was first described by patterson and kelly and later by Plummer and vinson.

It is usually seen in middle aged females

SYMPTOMS:
1. Dysphagia with severe attacks of retching.
2. The tongue is bald, is devoid of papillae associated with cheliosis.
3. The finger nails are brittle and are spoon shaped.
4. Spleen, is palpable.
5. There is evidence of Achlorhydria.
6. Blood shows Hypochromic anaemia.
7. Bone marrow is devoid of iron stores.

TREATMENT:
1. Correction of anaemia.
2. Dilatation of oesophageal stricture.

★ ★ ★ ★

9. NERVOUS SYSTEM

Q-1. Discuss motor Neurone disease. (1988 Supp.)

Ans. This is progressive chronic idiopathic degeneration of the motor neurones in the cerebral cortex, brain stem and spinal cord resulting in gradual atrophy, weakness, paralysis of muscles with fasiculations

Sensory and cerebellar dysfunctions are absent

AETIOLOGY: Unknown.

CLINICAL FEATURES:
1. ONSET: is insidious.
2. AGE: 40-60 yrs.
3. SEX: males are more affected.
4. CLINICAL TYPES: Following 3 types are seen:

a. PROGRESSIVE MUSCULAR ATROPHY: The lesion is chiefly located in the anterior horn cells.

There is usually non symmetrical wasting of small muscles of the hand which progresses centrally. The wasted muscles show marked fasiculation.

The interosseous spaces, thenar and Hypothenar eminences are hollowed out and gives the appearance of main en griffe hand.

The jerks are dull or lost and plantar is flexor in type. There are no sensory changes.

b. AMYOTROPHIC LATERAL SCLEROSIS: Here the lesion is not only in anterior horn cells but progresses to involve the pyramidal tracts.

Clinically it resembles the atrophic type but the jerks are exaggerated and the plantar becomes extensor.

In the upper limb the main features of lower motor neurone type i.e. wasting and fasciculations are seen but the jerks are brisk and the tone is increased.

In the lower limbs the features of upper motor neurone

lesion will dominate and therefore the reflexes are brisk, with increased tone and extensor plantar.

3. **PROGRESSIVE BULBAR PALSY:** The lesion is located in the medulla around the bulbar nuclei of the last 4 cranial nerves.

There is progressive weakness and wasting of tongue, palate, pharynx, lips and larynx giving rise to dysarthria, dysphagia, aphonia.

The mouth remains full of saliva and there is always an evidence of secondary infection.

PROGNOSIS: It is a disease with progressive course therefore the patient dies within 3-5 yrs of the period of disease.

Q-2. Describe poliomyelitis. Describe various methods to control the disease. Mention Homoeopathic medicines to treat it. (1976, 1982, 1988 Supp.)

Ans. **POLIOMYELITIS:** is an acute systemic disease caused by R.N.A virus which replicates mainly in the gastro intestinal tract. The virus reaches the central nervous system and damages the anterior Horn cells of spinal cord.

CLINICAL FEATURES:

1. **PRODROMAL STAGE:** It starts either with sore throat, coryza or cough or with vomiting, diarrhoea, constipation or with constitutional symptoms like malaise, fever, drowsiness, irritability.
2. **PREPARALYTIC STAGE:** In this phase the features of meningeal irritation are present.
a. Fever: Temperature rises to 39° c with pain and stiffness of back.
b. Moderate headache with nausea and vomiting.
c. Pains: are spontaneous evoked by movement of back, neck etc.
d. Hyperesthesia: either localised or generalised is present.
e. Rigidity in the neck and back are present.
f. Pulse is fast and out of proportion to rise of temperature.

g. The patient is always alert.
3. PARALYTIC STAGE: It usually develops between 2nd and 5th days after the onset of signs of involvement of nervous system.
    The features are
a. The symptoms appear while there is fever.
b. Distribution is asymmetrical.
c. The lower limbs are more frequently affected.
d. Respiratory disturbances due to involvement of diaphragm and accessory muscles.
4. CONVALESENCE: Initial phase of paralysis usually diminishes after a period of 2-3 wks. and improvement may continue for some months, when the chronic stage is reached six months to an year after initial infection, no further spontaneous improvement can be expected.

METHODS TO CONTROL THE DISEASE:
1. Isolation of infected cases.
2. Use of active Immunization: either by salk inactivated polio vaccine or Sabin oral live attenuated vaccine is given.
3. Passive Immunization: It is given according to the age of the child.

HOMOEOPATHIC MEDICINES.
1. STRYCHNINE: It is one of the best remedies for poliomyelitis. There is violent jerking, twitching and trembling of limbs with stiffness.

    There are cramp like pains with marked irritability in temperament

    All the complaints are worse in the morning, by touch, noise or by motion.
2. LATHYRUS: It usually affects the anterior and lateral colums of the spinal cord.

    The child cannot extend or cross legs when sitting. Stiffness and lameness of ankles and knees, toes do not leave the floor, heels do not touch the floor.

    He sits up in a bend forward posture and straightens up with difficulty.

    The reflexes are diminished.

3. KALI PHOS: It is suited to those persons who are weak prostrated both physically and mentally. There is marked prostration with great dread of doing any work.

There is paralytic weakness with lameness in back and extremities. Pains with depression and subsequent exhausation. Exertion aggravates.

Q-3. What is paraplegia? Give the causes, clinical features and treatment. (1980, 1987.)

Ans. Paralysis confined to the lower limbs is called paraplegia.

ETIOLOGY:
1. DEGENERATIVE DISEASES: Subacute combined degeneration, multiple sclerosis, Friedrich's ataxia.
2. TRAUMA: Fractures, dislocation of vertebral column.
3. INFECTIONS: Syphilis, Transverse myelitis.
4. VASCULAR: Haemorrhage and Thrombosis.
5. COMPRESSION: Spinal tumours, cervical spondylosis.
6. CHRONIC MALNUTRITION: Pellagra.
7. TOXINS: Lathyrism.
8. RADIATION: myelopathy.

CLINICAL FEATURES:
They can be discussed under the following heads:
1. MOTOR SYSTEM
a. Wasting in the presence of increased jerks is suggestive of Amyotrophic lateral sclerosis.
b. Coordination Ataxia is seen in S A C D of cord, multiple sclerosis.
c. Involuntary movements: Seen in A. Lateral sclerosis, multiple sclerosis.
2. SENSORY
a. Dissociated Anaesthesia seen in syringomyelia, Intra medullary tumours.
b. Total Loss of sensations: In complete cord transection
3. SPEECH
a. Stacto's speech: In multiple sclerosis, syringomyelia
b. Cranial Nerves: Nystagmus in multiple sclerosis, Pupillary changes in Syphilis.

4. REFLEXES: Knee jerk absent with absent ankle jerks with extensor plantar is seen in SA CD of cord.
5. SPHINCTERS: Usually loss of control is seen in multiple sclerosis, SACD of cord, cauda equinna lesions.
6. TROPHIC CHANGES: in Syringomyelia.

TREATMENT:
1. Correction of underlying cause.
2. Physiotherapy.
3. Surgery is also beneficial in some cases.
4. For further details See Q-8 of Excretory system.

Q-4. What is Bell's Palsy? What are the main findings on examination? Name 4 drugs. (1977, 1987.)

Ans. BELL'S PALSY: After exposure to cold, the patient complains of pain behind the ear, within a few hours notices inability to close the eye on the same side. It is Bell's Palsy.

CAUSES:
1. Exposure to cold.
2. Suppurative otitis media.
3. Herpes Zoaster.
4. Head Injury.

SYMPTOMS:
1. Sudden exposure to chills with or without any precipitating cause within 24 hrs leads to the development of it.
2. Pain behind the ear.
3. Spontaneously there is loss of taste, watering of eyes.and sweating is less on the affected side.

SIGNS ON EXAMINATION:
1. Forehead cannot be wrinkled, frowning is lost.
2. Eyes cannot be closed. On attempting closure, eyeball turns upwards and outwards (Bell's Phenomenon)
3. On showing the teeth, the lips do not separate on affected side whistling is not possible. Naso labial fold is flattened. Angle of mouth on affected side droops with dribbling of saliva.

Nervous System

4. Cheeks puff out with expiration because of paralysis of buccinator.
5. Food collects between teeth and paralysed cheek.

HOMOEOPATHIC MANAGEMENT:

1. **BELLADONA**: There is extreme congestion with severe throbbing headache. He does not want to move out of perpendicular position.

   Tingling sensation in affected parts better by cold applications. There is throbbing of carotids with extreme fear and excitablity.

2. **CADMIUM**: Numbness and coldness of affected parts. Wants to cover the affected area. Slightest exposure causes aggravation.

   Constipation, general malaise, restlessness along with increased coldness.

3. **STRAMONIUM**: It is chronic to Belladona. Symptoms of increased intensity with great senstivity, restlessness. All complaints are better after sleep.

4. **CAUSTICUM**: The pains are associated with numbness. The complaints usually develop in the females who are weepy, sympathetic and do not like to talk to any body, tearful and depressed.

   It is good for Right sided palsy when the complaints are aggravated in clear fine weather but better in damp weather.

Q-5. What are the causes of Hemiplegia? Discuss about cerebral Thrombosis and it's management. (1975 Supp, 1977 Supp, 1982, 1988 Supp.)

Ans. **CAUSES OF HEMIPLEGIA OF SUDDEN ONSET**
1. Vascular causes: Thrombosis, embolism, Haemorrhage
2. Intracranial infections like Meningitis, encephalitis.
3. Trauma.
4. Multiple sclerosis.
5. Hysterical.

OF SLOW ONSET
1. Cerebral Tumours.
2. Cerebral abscess.
3. General paralysis of insane.
4. Chronic subdural Haematoma.

CEREBRAL THROMBOSIS:

The formation of thrombus anywhere in the cerebral circulation is called cerebral Thrombosis.

ETIOLOGY:
1. Atherosclerosis.
2. Arteritis: Infective, giant cell arteritis.
3. Vasospasm.
4. Aneurysm of major or minor vessels.

CLINICAL FEATURES:
1. ONSET: The onset is usually sudden or progressive.
2. AGE: Commonly seen in middle aged or old people.
3. PREMONITARY SYMPTOMS: There is difficulty in speaking or weakness of arm or leg.
4. CLINICAL PRESENTATION:

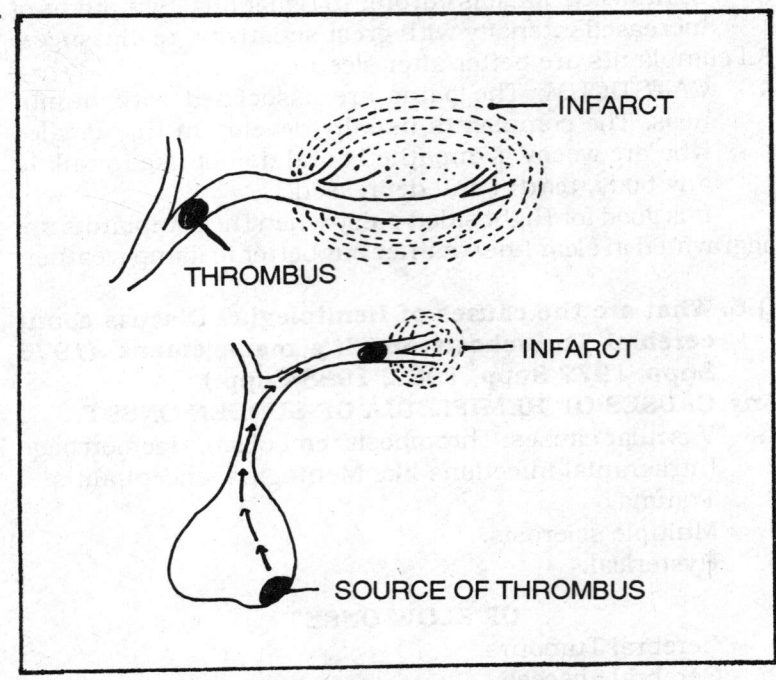

(CEREBRAL THROMBUS)

Nervous System

a. Headache is usually slight.
b. Vomiting at the onset is rare.
c. Convulsions are rare.
d. Coma: usually varies with the extent of thrombosis
e. Cheyne's stoke's Respiration: is rarely seen.
f. Bilateral extensor plantar may be present.
g. B.P is usually High.
5. C.S.F: is usually clear with slight raised pressure.
6. RECOVERY: is generally quick with no sequale.

MANAGEMENT:
The main principles are:
1. Restoration of Normal Systolic Blood pressure.
2. Adequate oxygenation.
3. Avoidance of Hypercapnia.
4. Abolition of Seizures.
5. Surgical Treatment: When the underlying cause is of orgin such that it requires surgical interference, then it should be undertaken.

Q-6. What is peripheral Neuropathy? What are the causes with signs and symptoms. Give 4 main drugs. (1987.)

Ans. PERIPHERAL NEUROPATHY: It is a clinical syndrome of multiple etiology which is characterised by impaired functioning of peripheral nerves resulting in the distribution of symmetrical flaccid weakness of mucles along with sensory changes affecting more the distal segments.

ETIOLOGY:
1. METABOLIC AND ENDOCRINE DISORDERS: Diabetes mellitus, gout., acromeagly
2. TOXINS AND DRUGS: alcohol, Isoniazid, Heavy metal poisoning
3. DEFICIENCY OF VITAMINS: Beriberi, Pellagra, vit B_{12} deficiency.
4. INFECTIONS: Diptheria, Tetanus, infective polyneuritis. leprosy.
5. MALIGNANCY: CA of lung.

SYMPTOMS AND SIGNS:
1. MOTOR CHANGES: Usually extensors are affected more then the flexors. There is atrophy of muscles with flaccidity. It may present as wrist or Foot drop.
2. SENSORY CHANGES:
a. Numbness, tingling, feeling of pins and needles with burning sensations, pain in extremities, sensation of walking in cotton wool with unsteadiness on walking.
3. AUTONOMIC DYSFUNCTIONS: Dryness or excessive sweating of extremities, postural Hypotension, impotence with sphincter disturbances.
4. TROPHIC CHANGES: Skin is glossy, coldness of extremities with falling of nails.

SIGNS:
1. SENSORY: a. Impairment of all sensations i.e. touch, pressure, temperature.
b. Tenderness of calf muscles.
c. Glove and stocking type of anaesthesia.
2. REFLEXES: Ankle jerk is the first to be affected. All the jerks are diminished or absent.

HOMOEOPATHIC DRUGS:
1. SECALE COR: The Knee jerk is completely absent. There is sensation as if feet are being dragged and is walking in air. He is unable to perform even light movements.

    There is sensation as of walking on a velvet.

    Gentle creeping sensation in the back as if soft air is blowing over it.

    Painful jerking of limbs particularly at night with lassitude, trembling and heaviness.

    The complaints are worse by heat and being covered.
2. PHYSOSTIGMA: There is constant feeling of unsteadiness on walking. Great weakness in legs below the Knees. must see where he is going. Always wants the support of a cane or a log when walking. Stiffness in Rectus femoris of thighs with great langour and flatulence and disturbed vision.
3. ONOSMODIUM: Tired, cold, numb feeling in the legs mostly below the knees. Gait is usually disturbed while

Nervous System

walking. Loss of muscular coordination with staggering gait.

Cannot keep concentration of mind, must think constantly from changing topics There is a sense of formication in the calf muscles.

4. DUBIOSIN: It is indicated when the typical gait is present. It is almost impossible for the patient to stand with eyes closed.

Constant swaying in forward or backward direction. Sensation as if the floor is coming near to him specially when walking with eyes closed and taking high steps. Feels as if walking on empty space.

There is a sensation as if he could not hold his body up and will fall.

Tired, feeling with paralysis of accomodation and vertigo.

Q-7. Differentiate epileptic fit from hysteria. How would you treat a child of 5 yrs having repeated attacks of epilepsy? Describe 3 drugs for petit mal epilepsy. (1977 W. Bengal, 1974 Supp, 1975 Supp, 1980, 1982, 1987 Supp, 1992.)

Ans. EPILEPSY	HYSTERIA
1. The attack has a constant periodicity.	It is induced by emotional excitement.
2. Incontinence is common	No incontinence.
3. Tongue biting with injury from fall.	Not seen.
4. It can occur anywhere.	usually in the presence of people.
5. Tonic and clonic phases.	There are spectacular movements.
6. Ext plantar response.	Not extensor.
7. Corneal Reflex is absent during the attack.	It is present.
8. Conjugate deviation of head and eyes.	No turning of head and eyes, eyeballs roll upwards
9. Attacks of short duration.	It may be prolonged.
10. Gradual recovery.	Recovery is sudden.

MANAGEMENT:
1. General hygiene and Diet, regular habits of eating and sleeping, adequate Diet.
2. Correction of worm Infestation: by Deworming treatment
3. Use of Antiepileptic drugs.

HOMOEOPATHIC DRUGS:
1. ARTEMESIA VULGARIS: The child is very irritable, depressed with vexation just a day before the attack. Attacks generally occur at night. Violent emotions usually precipitate the attack.

   Few attacks come in repetition with a period free from the attack.

   Left pupil is more dilated then the Right at the time of attack.

   They are unconscious only for few seconds when they are busy in their works.
2. ASTERIAS RUBENS: It is useful in focal epilepsy when several days before the attack there is twitching of muscles. During this period she is irritable, restless with pallor of the face.

   Attacks come suddenly with movements of the jaw. It can be used for Hallucinations of attack; feels as if he is away from home, or in midst of strangers or hears noises distantly.
3. OENANTHE CROCATA: There are facial twitchings with lividity of face. After the attack the pulse is increased.

   The attacks are associated with nausea, vomiting and vertigo with a feeling of heat in the stomach. Eyes are turned upwards with dilated pupils. Attacks generally occur at night.

Q-8. Discuss the etiology, clinical features with Homoeopathic treatment of Locomotor ataxia. (1978 Supp, 1982, 1983.)
Ans. Difficulty in walking is called Ataxia.

ETIOLOGY :
1. CEREBELLAR ATAXIA

Nervous System   149

a. cerebellar tumour, abscess, cerebellar artery thrombosis.
b. Friedrich's Ataxia
2. SENSORY ATAXIA
a. Peripheral Neuritis.
b. Posterior Root affections like. Tabes Dorsalis.
c. Post Column: multiple Sclerosis, Syringomyelia.
3. LABYRINTHINE ATAXIA:
a. Acute labyrinthitis.
b. Haemorrhage into internal ear.
c. Meniere's Disease.

CLINICAL FEATURES
1. Age of onset is usually 10-30 yrs.
2. There is truncal ataxia with ataxia of lower limbs with a reeling gait.
3. Gradually the upper limbs are also involved.
4. Dysarthria with lost jerks and Extensor plantar is seen.
6. Muscular Hypotonia is also present.
7. Associated Abnormalities: Pes cavus, kyphosis or Kyphoscolosis are seen.

FOR HOMOEOPATHIC DRUGS: See Q-6.

Q-9. Describe various types of CVA. Give the salient features with their distinguishing points. (1990, 1991)

Ans. The term CVA usually implies the development of focal disturbances in cerebral functions due to vascular causes.

They can be classified into:
1. Cerebral Ischaemic disease of arterial origin
a. Transient ischaemic attacks.
b. Progressing stroke
c. Completed stroke
2. Venous Infarct
3. Subarachnoid Haemorrhage

		EMBOLISM	THROMBOSIS	HAEMORRHAGE
1.	Age	young.	middle or old.	middle age or old.
2.	Nature of onset	Instantaneous.	Sudden or progressive.	Catastrophic. usually absent.

3.	Premonitary Symptoms	Absent	Difficulty in speaking, weakness in arm or leg.	
4.	Common cause	M.S with atrial fibrilation, carotid stenosis.	Areriosclerosis with or without HT.	Hypertension is always present.
5.	Clinical Features			
1.	Headache	variable.	slight or absent.	severe.
2.	Vomiting	Rare.	Rare.	Common.
3.	Convulsions	Common.	Rare.	common.
4.	Coma	Rarely deep.	Varies with the extent of Thrombosis.	Deep unconsciousness
5.	Cheyne's stokes Respiration	Not Common.	Seldom.	Common.
6.	Stiffness of Neck	Rare	Rare.	Frequent.
7.	Conjugate deviation of eyes	Rare.	Seldom.	Frequent.
8.	B/L extensor plantar	Rare.	may be present.	Frequent.
9.	Reaction of pupil to light	No change	may be Impaired.	usually impaired.
10.	B.P	Normal.	may be high	usually high.
11.	C.S.F	usually (N).	clear with slight increased in pressure.	usually bloody with increased pressure.
6.	CAT SCAN	Infarction may not apear for 2-4 days.	same.	can be confirmed within minutes of onset.
7.	TERMINATION	Recovery is usual.	Recovery often.	High mortality.

Q-10. What are the causes of sudden Hemiplegia? Discuss the Differential Diagnosis with Homoeopathic Remedies. (1974, 1976, 1985)

Ans. CAUSES OF SUDDEN HEMIPLEGIA:

1. Vascular causes: Embolism, Thrombosis etc.
2. Post epileptic paralysis.
3. Trauma-depressed fracture.
4. Intracraninal infections: Encephalitis, meningitis.

Nervous System

5. Hypertensive encephalopathy.
6. Multiple sclerosis.
7. Hysterical.
8. Uraemia.

For DD See Q-9 Chart.

HOMOEOPATHIC MEDICINES:

1. LATHYRUS SATIVUS: See Q-2.
2. CURARE WOORARI: Debility after loss of fluids or exhausting illnesses. It is good for (R) sided paralysis specially in aged. Eyes give a look of being sunken and depressed.

   The complaints are worse by the change of weather and from cold drinks.

3. SILLICEA: Paralysis from defective nutrition of nervous system. Brain and spine cannot bear ordinary vibration or concussion. Skin is tender and sensitive to touch.

   Paralysis resulting as a sequale of convulsions. It is helpful in DYSPHAGIA PARALYTICA. Paralysis of left side of both arm and leg with atrophy and numbness.

   Along with paralysis there is heaviness of head, ringing in ears, great debility, wants to lie down all the time. Limbs go to sleep very frequently.

   Limbs are sore and cold with trembling as if they have lost all the power.

   All the complaints are from suppressed Foot Sweat. It should be given in low potencies.

Q-11. What are Demyelinting Disease? Discuss any one in detail. (1989.)

Ans. These are the group of diseases which have some clinical and pathological features in common. The most important change is the loss of myelin sheath with minimum or no damage to axis cylinder. The nature of these diseases is uncertain.

They include:
1. Acute Disseminated encephalo myelitis.
2. Acute Haemorrhagic Leuco encephalomyelitis.
3. multiple sclerosis.
4. Neuro myelitis optica.

5. Diffuse cerebral sclerosis.

MULTIPLE SCLEROSIS

It is the commonest of all demyelinating diseases.

ETIOLOGY:

Exact cause is unknown. It has a definite genetic linkage.

Excessive consumption of animal fat may held to be responsible.

PATHOLOGY: Demyelination occurs in different places and at different phases of the disease white plaques are formed in the white matter of C.N.S.

The most common sites are
1. Cervical spinal cord
2. Brain stem with cerebellum
3. Periventricular region
4. Optic Nerves.

CLINICAL FEATURES:

1. AGE: Between 15-50 yrs.
2. SEX: Both sexes are equally affected.
3. PRECIPITATING FACTORS: like infections, trauma, emotional upsets or fatigue are responsible.
4. PSYCHOLOGICAL SYMPTOMS: In the form of mood changes, depression are very common.
5. OCULAR SYMPTOMS: Unilateral Retro bulbar neuritis is the earliest manifestation. Double vision, nystagmus, swelling of optic disc, with temporal pallor are seen.
6. MOTOR SYMPTOMS: include hemiplegia, monoplegia, intention tremors, scanning speech.
7. SENSORY SYMPTOMS: Tingling, numbness, impaired postural sense, electric shock like pains are seen.
8. REFLEXES: Abdominal Reflexes are lost early plantars become extensor.
   sphincters are affected in the later stage.
9. PAROXYSMAL SYMPTOMS: like Trigeminal neuralgia, spasms with dysarthria, ataxia are seen.

TREATMENT: No specific treatment but use of GABA derivatives is useful. But Homoeopathic medicines like Causticum, Zincum Phos, Phosphorus, Plumbum met can be used on the basis of totality.

Nervous System

Q-12. Discuss the D.D of coma. How will you manage such a case? Mention 3 Homoeopathic medicines with indications. (1977)
Ans. CAUSES OF COMA:

1. BRAIN STEM LESIONS a. Infarction b. Pontine Haemorrhage c. Cerebellar Haematoma d. Tumours e. Secondary effects of mass lesion in Cerebral Hemisphere.	Rapid onset of coma. Pupils are fixed with abnormal light response Pinpoint pupils Cranial Nerve Signs Long Tract Signs
2. SUPRA TENTORIAL MASS LESIONS a. Cerebral Haemorrhage b. Space occupying Lesions c. massive cerebral Infarction.	Signs of causations lesion Brain stem lesion signs due to compression.
3. METABOLIC CAUSES a. Anoxia b. Respiratory failure c. Wernickes Encephalopathy	Absence of Signs of focal lesion in CNS. Pupillary response is preserved Cheyne' stoke's Resp is present. Eye movements are full and conjugate.
4. DIFFUSE INTRACRANICAL DISORDERS a. Head Injury b. meningitis c. Epilepsy d. H.T encephalopathy e. Subarachnoid Haemorrhage	See chart for Diff of CVA.

For management: See Q-9 of Excretory system

HOMOEOPATHIC MEDICINES:
1. OPIUM: It is one of the best medicines for coma. There

is complete loss of consciousness with apoplexy.

Face is red, bloated dark, suffused and hot with warm sweat.

Pulse is full and slow with irregular respiration. There is incontinence of stool and urine.

There is hot perspiration all over the body except lower limbs.

2. AMYL NITRATE: It causes dilatation of all arterioles, capillaries producing flushings of face with heat and throbbing of all vessels. There is great oppression and fullness of chest with tumultous action of the heart.
3. PILOCARPINE: Pulse is irregular, dicrotic with cyanosis and oppression of chest. Pupils are small and contracted. There is constant dribbling of saliva from the mouth. The eyes give a staring wide look. Slow sighing Respiration.

Q-13. What are the diseases of Lower motor Neurome. Describe the complications of one of these diseases including its management. (1980.)

Ans. The diseases of LMN are:
1. Poliomyelitis
2. Tabes Dorsalis
3. Cauda Equinna Syndrome
4. Fried rich's Ataxia
5. Motor Neurone disease.

COMPLICATIONS OF POLIOMYELITIS:
1. Respiratory Failure.
2. Hypotension.
3. Cardiovascular Failure.

MANAGEMENT:
1. PREPARALYTIC STAGE
a. Rest in bed.
b. Sedation
c. Heat in the form of moist packs in relieving muscle soreness.
2. PARALYTIC STAGE
a. Splints for paralysed muscles
b. Physiotherapy.

Nervous System

c. maintainence of fluid intake with proper dietary intake.
d. Catheterisation.
e. Use of Enemas if abdominal muscles are weak.
f. maintenance of Respiration.
3. CONVALESCENT STAGE:
a. Physiotherapy.
b. Muscle re-education.
c. Application of appropriate Corrective appliances.
d. Orthopaedic surgery.
e. Rehabilitation of severly paralysed children.

Q-14. A child aged about 4 yrs is brought to you with convulsions. How do you manage the case Suggest 4 Homoeopathic Remedies. (1983, 1984.)

Ans. See Q-7.

Q-15. Describe the clinical features of epilepsy. (1974, 1977.)

Ans. The clinical features can be described according to the type of epilepsy.
1. **GRAND MAL EPILEPSY:**

PRODROMAL PHASE

There is uneasiness, irritability hours or days before the attack.

AURA:

Due to partial onset of seizure it lasts for seconds or minutes eg : olfactory hallucinations, epigastric discomfort, jerking of one limb.

TONIC PHASE

There is rapid discharging of impulse from motor cortex cells which causes tonic contractions of muscles.
a. Arms flexed and adducted with extension of legs.
b. Respiratory muscle spasm causes CRY as air is expelled.
c. Cyanosis.
d. Loss of consciousness lasting for 10-30 Seconds.

CLONIC PHASE

There is less rapid, gradually slowing, discharge from cortex cells.

a. There is violent jerking of face and limbs, biting of tongue, Incontinence of faeces or urine.
b. Choking due to accumalation of Secretions

This phase lasts for 1-5 min.

POST ICTAL PHASE
1. Deep unconsciousness, with flaccidity of jaw and limbs.
2. Loss of corneal reflex.
3. Extensor plantar response
4. Headache, Confusion, aching muscles and sometimes automatic behaviour, ocasional violence.

2. **PETIT MAL EPILEPSY:** It is an uncommon form of epilepsy mostly seen in children.
   a. **Typical abscences** are seen in the form of stares, may blink the eyes, stops the activity, failure to respond to command.
   b. **Akinetic seizures:** There is loss of posture and the child falls but is able to get up again quickly.
3. **FOCAL EPILEPSY:** It is due to localised irritation of motor cortex.

It can be seen in the following forms:
1. MOTOR: Ther is rythmical jerking of arms, legs or any part which is localised to begin with but becomes generalised.
2. SENSORY: It is seen in the form of tingling or electric sensations in the contralateral face and limbs.
3. VERSIVE: It involves the frontal eye field causing forced deviation of the eyes to the opposite side.
4. VISUAL: Occipital epileptic foci, causes simple visual hallucinations such as balls of light or pattern of colour.
5. PSYCHOMOTOR: They are seen in the form of changes of mood, memory and perception. The phenomenon of undue familarity (Dejavu's) or unreality (Jamais vu) are seen.

There can be complex hallucinations of sound, smell, taste or vision.

Q-16. Give the Differential diagnosis and management of status epilepticus. (1978, 1983, 1991 Supp.)

Ans. DIFFERENTIAL DIAGNOSIS:
1. CONGENITAL CEREBRAL DEFECTS
a. Hydrocephalus.
b. Congenital Diaplegia.

2. HEAD INJURIES
a. Birth Trauma.

3. INTRACRANIAL INFECTIONS
a. meningitis   b. Cerebral malaria.
c. Encephalitis.
d. T.B.
4. GENERAL INFECTIONS
a. Gastroenteritis.
b. Otitis media.
c. Specific fevers.
d. Osteomyelitis.
5. INTOXICATIONS
a. Uraemia.
b. Poisons.
6. CEREBRAL TUMOURS
a. Primary Tumours.
b. Secondary metastasis.
7. CARDIOVASCULAR DISORDERS
a. Cerebral Thrombosis.
b. Paroxysmal fibrillation..
c. Hypertensive enceplalopathy.
8. Hysteria.
9. Idiopathic.
10. Carotid Sinus epilepsy.

MANAGEMENT OF STATUS EPILEPTICUS:
1. Adequate Respiratory Exchange. Institute oral suction and provide an airway by supporting the jaws in an extended position or by inserting an oral airway.
2. B. Pressure is to be watched closely.
3. Complete analysis for blood count, electrolytes and blood gas analysis.
4. Protection from External injuries by providing padding about the joints.
5. Drugs: Use of Anti epileptic drugs.

6. General Anaesthesia when all other steps are unsuccessful.

Q-17. Describe the clinical features and complications of Encephalitis. Mention 3 Homoeopathic drugs. (1981 Supp.)

Ans. **DEFINITION:** Acute inflammation of the brain and spinal cord caused by viral infection is called Encephalitis.

ETIOLOGY:
1. Acute Diseminated Encephalomyelitis: It is associated with enterovirses like Herpes simplex, Herpes Zoaster, varicella etc.
2. Post Infection Encephalo myelitis: following measles and vaccination, chickenpox etc.

CLINICAL FEATURES:
1. ONSET: is insidious with prodromal symptoms. There may be evidence of primary infection in the background.
2. CONSTITUTIONAL SYMPTOMS: Varies from mild indisposltion to profound toxic state. General body aches, pains headache and vomiting are common.
3. MENTAL SYMPTOMS: Restlessness is the earliest feature with impaired consciousness, delirium and a change in normal behaviour.
   Epileptic fits may also occur in few patients.
4. RESPIRATORY CHANGES: It is seen in the form of irregular respirations.
5. MANIFESTATIONS OF CNS:
a. Neck stiffness with Kernig's sign is present.
b. Focal signs include pupillary changes, ocular palsies, nystagmus, ataxia and Hemiplegia.
6. SPINAL CORD INVOLVEMENT: It is seen in later stages with paraplegia or with retention of urine.

COMPLICATIONS:
1. Parkinsonism
2. Respiratory Failure
3. Degeneration of cerebral cortex.

Nervous System

4. Deafness
5. Vestibular damage.

FOR HOMOEOPATHIC TREATMENT: See Q-2.

Q-18. A middle aged man while working in an office suddenly becomes unconscious. How would you investigate and make a differential diagnosis? Give 3 Homoeopathic medicines. (1977 Supp.)

Ans. Impairment of consicousness by injury, disease or intoxication may produce changes in behaviour which may be the outcome af alterations in the level of awareness.

The following conditions should be thought of

1. PETIT MAL EPILEPSY: In this attacks of absences usually occur 10-12/day. In this the person becomes awkward gives a vacant look with staring eyes. Within few seconds he recovers.
2. HYPOGLYCAEMIA: It is seen in persons who used Insulin indiscreminately in cases of D.M.

   The patient before becoming unconscious C/o hunger pains, general weakness, vertigo with dimness of vision.

   He immediately responds to glucose given orally.
3. HYSTERIA: Usually females are affected. The patient usually in the presence of public or family members becomes a subject of unconsciousness. No organic feature of any lesion is found on examination.
4. CAROTID SINUS SYNDROME: They usually result from overactivity of carotid sinus. It is associated with arteriosclerosis and Hypertension.
5. CEREBRAL SYNCOPE: It is a consequence of direct brain damage secondary to trauma or assoicated with vertebrobasilar disease. The attacks ocur in the errect posture.
6. POSTURAL SYNCOPE: It occurs as a result of failure of baroreceptors which normally adjust the heart rate and peripheral Resistence.
a. Arising abruptly from a prolonged period in recumbent position.
b. Following sternous exercise.
c. Chronic Orthostatic Hypotension.

INVESTIGATIONS:
1. Good clinical History itself is diagnostic.
2. Urine test.
3. Blood sugar, T.L.C, D.L.C, ESR.
4. E.E.G.
5. Adequate information from relatives.

For 3rd part See Q-12.

Q-19. Write short notes on
1. muscular Dystrophy (1975 Supp, 1985)
2. Sciatica (1978, 1985)
3. Writer's cramps (1983)
4. Argyll Robertson pupil (1974 Supp, 1974, 1975 Supp, 1976, 1977, 1983.)
5. Huntigton's chorea (1991 Supp.)
6. Lumbar puncture (1991 Supp)
7. Cerebral Aneurysm (1992.)
8. Flaccid paralysis (1978)
9. Hemiplegia (1978 Supp)
10. migraine (1978 Supp)
11. Coma vigil (1974 Supp)
12. Kerning's Sign. (1974 Supp)
13. Knee Jerk (1974 Supp)
14. Romberg's Sign (1975 Supp, 1980)
15. Babinski's sign (1975 Supp, 1980, 1981 Supp, 1982)
16. Chorea (1975 Supp, 1980, 1981 Supp)
17. Festinent gait (1976, 1977)
18. Charcot's Triad (1976, 1977)
19. Parkinsonism (1981 Supp)
20. Wernicke's Encephalopathy (1992)
21. Ankle clonus (1982)
22. Scanning speech (1983)
23. Spastic gait (1983)
24. Syndrome Guillian Barre (1983 supp.)

1. **MUSCULAR DYSTROPHY:** They are the group of diseases characterised by degeneration of muscles.

   They are usually genetic in nature with autosomal dominant character.

   AGE AND SEX: It usually affects the males of 5-15 yrs of age. Females are the carriers.

CLINICAL FEATURES:
1. ONSET: is gradual. From childhood it becomes manifested with difficulty in walking with late learning to walk.
2. ATTITUDE ON STANDING: There is marked lordosis of lumbar spine.
3. GAIT: There is typical waddling gait.
4. MUSCLES: usually there is symmetrical involvement of deltoid, glutei, quadriceps group of muscles with atrophy of muscles of upper limbs and those of glutei.
5. GOWER'S SIGN: is usually positive.

TYPES:
1. Duchene's Type
2. Limb girdle type
3. Fascioscapulo Humoral type.

PROGNOSIS: is bad and the child usually dies because of infections.

2. **SCIATICA:** Pain along the distribution of Sciatic nerves is called SCIATICA

ETIOLOGY:
1. Compression of spinal cord by tumours, cauda equinna or by haemorrhages.
2. In the Diseases of verrebral column: T.B of spine, Ankylosing spondylitis, Arthritis etc.
3. Neuritic disorders like Leprosy, S.L.E. Polyarteritis nodosa.

SYMPTOMS:
1. Onset is usually related to past dated trauma, exposure to cold or damp weather or even previous attacks.
2. There is severe pain in the direction of one or both the sciatic nerves which is made worse by coughing, sneezing or even by pressure.
3. The pain is associated with numbness in the distribution of nerve.
4. Associated Symptoms: Painful Tender heels, cramps in calves.

SIGNS:
1. SLR TEST: is +ve

2. Intensification of pain in back and leg during rotatory extension of lumbar spine.
3. Popliteal compression: also causes pain in the distribution of nerve.

TREATMENT:
1. Complete Rest in bed.
2. Use of analgesics
3. Use of injections via the epidural route.
4. Use of physiotherapy and Traction.
5. Homoeopathic Drugs like colocynth, Dioscorea and gnaphallium can be tried.

3. **WRITER'S CRAMPS:** It is a disorder of cerebral origin and consists of spasms and cramp like pain in the affected muscles when writing is attempted. It affects the adults usually those who write with intrinsic hand musles only, not from elbows or shoulder.

The onset of spasm and cramp like pain produces great ataxia in the writing. The writing becomes smaller and indecipherable.

TREATMENT.
1. Absolute Rest is essential.
2. Training to use (L) Land.
3. Reeducation with the use of large pen.
4. **ARGYLL ROBERTSON PUPIL:** It is a characteristic manifestation of Neurosyphilis. It has the following features.
1. Miosis generally bilateral.
2. Irregular pupils
3. Do not react to light
4. Reaction to accomodation is instantaneous.
5. Failure of pupils to dilate to painful stimuli.

CAUSES:
1. Tabes Dorsalis   5. Chronic alcohlism
2. General Paralysis of Insane 6. Brain stem Encephalitis
3. Multiple Sclerosis 7. Syringomyelia
4. Diabetes
5. **HUNTINGTONS CHOREA:** It is one of the commonest

Nervous System

extrapyramidal disorder of hereditary origin. It is also called chronic progressive chorea. It starts in the middle age with choreiform movements and progressive dementia. The rigid form may simulate PARKINSONISM.

ETIOLOGY:
It is due to the degeneration of ganglion cells of forebrain and corpus striatum.

6. **LUMBAR PUNCTURE:** It is one of the important diagnostic and therapeutic techniques used in Neurology.

   SITE: It is done between L_3 and L_4 vertebrae.

   NEEDLE USED: Vim Silverman or manghini's needle is used.

   DIAGNOSTIC INDICATIONS:
   1. For examination of C.S.F in unexplained coma, meningitis, Subarachnoid Haemorrhage.
   2. **THERAPEUTIC INDICATIONS:**
      a. Raised intracranial tension in Hypertensive encephalopathy.
      b. For introduction of drugs like antibiotics or steroids.
   3. For Anaesthesia.

   ### CONTRAINDICATIONS:
   1. markedly raised intracranial pressure as seen in papilloedema.
   2. Local gross spinal lesion and obvious neurological damage, because of fear of developing complete TRANSVERSE LESION.

7. **CEREBRAL ANEURYSM:** The dilatation of one of the cerbral arteries is called aneurysm

   ### CLINICAL FEATURES:
   1. Severe Headache usually worse in the morning on waking up not relieved by analgesics.
   2. Features of papilloedema and visual disturbances.
   3. Focal signs in the form of epilepsy
   4. When it bursts it causes Subarachnoid haemorrhage thereby causing hemilplegia, paraplegia.

8. **FLACCID PARALYSIS:** See Q-6
9. **HEMIPLEGIA:** See Q-5.

10. **MIGRAINE:** A paroxysmal disorder of cerebral function commonly assoicated with visual disturbances, unilateral headache and vomiting is called migraine.

ETIOLOGY:
1. AGE: It usually starts in the adolesence with progressively increasing attacks in adulthood.
2. SEX: more common in women.
3. PRECIPITATING CAUSES: Prolonged fasting, exposure to bright light, ingestion of amino acids in large amount.

CLINICAL FEATURES:
1. PRODROMAL SYMPTOMS: They usually last for 15-20 minutes before the headache. They are related either to vision in the form of light scintillations or to sensory phenomenon in the form of numbness and paresthesiae in face.
2. CLASSICAL HEADACHE: It may be hemicrania but soon becomes generalised. It starts with vague pain but soon becomes throbbing in intensity associated with pallor, nausea, vomiting and photophobia. It may last for several hours and is decreased after vomiting.

TREATMENT:
1. Use of analgesics.
2. Lying in a dark and quiet room with ice. pack on the head may be beneficial.
3. Homoeopathic Remedies like Natmur, Sanguinaria, Spigelia, onosmodium etc can be used.

11. **COMA VIGIL:** In coma patient gets up, opens his eyes and turns his head from side to side as if examining his enviroment.

In coma, final stage of recovery is marked by return of the capacity to recall current events with correct orientation and insight.

12. **KERNING'S SIGN:** The presence of neck rigidity in any kind of intracranial infections is called kernig's sign.

HOW TO ELICIT: Ask the patient to sit straight. If there is doubt of meningeal irritation then gradually the neck is bent and allowed to touch the sternum. If it is touched without any pain or stiffness being felt then it is -ve. But if the stiffness is felt then the sign is +ve.

It becomes evident in
1. Meningitis
2. Meningism
3. Spasm of Neck muscles from which it can be clinically differentiated.
13. **KNEE JERK:** The innervation of the Knee joint muscles is by L_2 L_3 and at times by L_4 dermatomes. Therefore the root value of this jerk is L_2 L_3 L_4.

HOW TO ELICIT: Ask the patient to sit on the chair with extended leg. Now ask him to relax it completely. Strike the narrow end of the hammer keeping a finger on the point of tibial tuberosity.

ABSENT KNEE JERKS:
1. Infective Polyneuritis
2. Peripheral Neuritis
3. Progressive muscular atrophy.
4. Muscle dystrophy
5. Acute Transverse myelitis.

EXAGGERATED JERKS:
1. Motor Neurone Disease
2. Upper motor Neurone Lesion
3. Multiple Sclerosis.

14. **ROMBERG'S SIGN:** It is usually done to elicit the functioning or any kind of abnormality of posterior column.

Ask the patient to stand with feet close to each other. Now ask him to close the eyes and stand.

The physcian keeps his both hands on the side of the patient as to support him.

The patient when tends to fall on either side is supported by the physcian. Then the test is considered to be positive.

15. **BABINSKI'S SIGN:** The plantar response when elicited in infants shows extension of big toe with fanning out of the small toes. It is called Babinski's sign.

In the infants upto 1 yr it is considered to be Normal.

INDICATIONS: When present in adult it usually indicates

1. Upper motor Neurore type of Lesion
2. motor neutone disease
3. Very rarely it is considered to be Normal in anxious personalities.
   It is innerated by $L5_1$ S and S_2.
16. **CHOREA:** See part 5 of Q-19.
17. **FESTINENT GAIT:** It is also called SHORT.
    SHUFFLING GAIT. It is usually seen in Extrapyramidal lesions specially in Parkinsonism.
    The patient is seen in a bent posture taking small steps due to rigidity; with instability and lack of confidence.
    Although he is walking slowly but it appears that he is running and is running fast, after his centre of gravity.
    The patient usually finds difficulty in taking a turn and when given a push he tends to fall.
18. **CHARCOT'S TRIAD:** The triad of Nystagmus in the Horizontal plane, with intention tremors and Stacto's speech due to Cerebellar involvement is called Charcot's triad.
    1. SPEECH: The words are spoken syllable by syllable.
    2. INTENTION TREMORS: The fine tremors usually occur when intends to do anything. But disappear when at rest.
    3. NYSTAGMUS: It develops in the lateral gaze particulary towards the side of lesion.
19. PARKINSONISM: It is one of the commonest of all extrapyramidal disorders.

ETIOLOGY:
1. Idiopathic or Parkinsonism or primary.
2. Secondary to
a. Wilson's Disease.
b. Encephalitis.
c. Toxins.
d. Alcohlism.

CLINICAL FEATURES:
1. It is seen in elderly males of 40-50 yrs of life.
2. It starts with slowness of all activities; he cannot fasten

up the buttons or he cannot do fast enough in daily routine.
3. Appearance: There is greasy look of face with a staring vacant appearance.
4. Tremors or Pill Rolling movements are constantly seen at Rest.
5. Short Shuffling gait.
6. Lead pipe type of Rigidity in Extremities with Normal Reflexes.
7. **GLABELLAR TAP TEST:** is usually positive
1. Senile Tremors   **D D**
2. Arteriosclerosis
3. Toxic Tremors.
20. **WERNICKE'S ENCEPHALOPATHY:** The deficiency of vit B_1 resulting in petechial haemorrhages in the midbrain and mamillary bodies leads to the clinical presentation of wernicke's encephalopathy.

CLINICAL FEATURES:
1. Rapidly coming mental confusion with disorientation of time and place.
2. Increasing but restless sleep which advances to coma.
3. Signs show ophthalmic disturbances causing restricted movements of eyeball, nystagmus, drooping of eyelids with abnormal pupillary reflexes.
4. Plantar reflex is extensor with features of cerebellar ataxia in the limbs.
21. **ANKLE CLONUS:** It is best elicited with the patient on his back with hip slightly abducted, thigh slightly rotated externally hip and knee slightly flexed.

This position is maintained with one hand under the thigh while with the other hand the foot is rapidly dorsiflexed and is held in position by even pressure.

It always indicates DAMAGE TO PYRAMIDAL TRACTS. It can also be seen in Nervous persons ocasionally.
22. **SCANNING SPEECH:** The violent, jerky and explosive speech of cerebellar dysfunction is called scanning speech.

In this type the words are spoken syllable by syllable like Artillery as A-A-R T1 - LE - RRy.

It is an important component of CHARCOT'S TRIAD.

23. **SPASTIC GAIT:** It is generally seen in spastic paraplegia where the patient moves swiftly along with abnormally short steps, the front part of the foot clinging to the ground produced by bilateral circumduction of the legs.

In severe cases tendency to ankle clonus causes a trepidiation of the whole body from tremors of the feet.

24. **GUILLAIN BARRE SYNDROME:** It is also called acute Idiopathic polyneuritis.

ETIOLOGY:

1. AGE: usually between 20-50 yrs with male predominance

CLINICAL FEATURES See peripheral neuropathy See Q.6

25. Compare meningococcal and T.B Meningitis

MENINGOCOCCAL MENINGITIS	T.B MENINGITIS
1. ETIOLOGY: It is caused by meningococcal meningitides.	It is caused by Acid fast Mycobacterium T.B.
2. It is usually seen in children and adolesents.	It is seen in middle aged persons.
3. ONSET: is sudden and dramatic.	It is usually insidious with low grade fever and cachexia.
4. C.S.F CHANGES a. It is turbid. b. Sugar is markedly reduced. c. Cells: Polymorphs are seen. d. Culture: Shows microrganisms with other associated Cocci.	clear or slightly opaque It is very mildly reduced. Lymphocytes are seen. It shows only mycobacterium T.B.

★ ★ ★ ★

10. RESPIRATORY SYSTEM

Q-1. What is lung abscess? Discuss the Differential diagnosis, general management and Homoeopathic drugs to treat this condition (1988.)

Ans. DEFINITION: Circumscribed suppurative inflammation of the lung tissue by pyogenic organisms leading to cavitation and Necrosis, is lung abscess **D.D:**

1. BRONCHIECTASIS: There is history of cough influenced by posture associated with copious sputum. X-Ray shows the characteristic dilatations of terminal bronchioles with prominent Bronchovesicular markings.
2. EMPYEMA WITH BRONCHO PLEURAL FISTULA: The fistula can be demonstrated by injecting 2 ml of 1% methylene blue into the empyema and examining the sputum for dye.
3. INFECTED LUNG CYSTS: particularly the bronchogenic and Hydatid cysts get infected Radiological evidence shows the presence of clear cut spherical shadow with little or no surrounding pneumonitis.
4. CAVITATED BRONCHIAL CA: The patient is elderly with pain in chest, cough, dyspnoea and other pressure symptoms. Enlarged axillary or cervical glands are found with cytological evidence of cells in the sputum.
5. PULMONARY INFARCT: It is seen either post operative or with an antecedent cardiovascular disease. The sputum is always blood stained with the presence of friction rub. X-Ray shows a wedge shaped consolidation.
6. CYSTIC FIBROSIS: There is a symptom complex of

pancreatic insufficiency, chronic pulmonary infection with High sodium content of the sweat.
7. WEIGNER'S GRANULOMATOSIS: Respiratory symptoms like cough, Haemoptysis, dyspnoea are present with radiological evidence of lesions in both the lower lung fields. Cavitation is seen with sharply outlined borders and thin walls.

MANAGEMENT:
1. GENERAL:
   a Rest in bed.
   b. High caloric. High protein diet with additional vitamins
   c. Deep breathing exercises to encouerage drainage
2. MECHANICAL PROCEDURES:
   a. Postural Drainage
   b. Bronchoscopic suction
   c. O_2 inhalations if the sputum is foul smelling
3. CHEMOTHERAPY: The use of antibiotics.
4. SURGICAL RESECTION: If within a period of 3-4 weeks there is no improvement, surgical resection is done.

HOMOEOPATHIC TREATMENT
1. BACILLINUM: It is very useful when the underlying cause is of tubercular origin. It is indicated in chest affections with feeble pulmonary circulation and attacks of suffocation at night. There is excessive bringing up of foul smelling sputum.
2. BALSAM PERU: It is a very good remedy for Bronchial catarrh when the sputum is thick, creamy and mucopurulent in nature. Very loose cough with loud rales in the chest. Hectic fever with nocturnal sweats.
3. STANNUM METALLICUM: The mucus is expelled by forcible cough. Cough is excited by laughing singing, talking and worse lying on (R) side.

While coughing lot of greenish sweetish expectoration is brought up. The chest always feels weak and sore with Nocturnal sweats.

Q-2. Describe Bronchial Asthma with the complications

Respiratory System

and treatment in detail. Mention about the status Asthmaticus. (1974, 1977, 1974 Supp, 1975 Supp, 1978, 1982, 1988 Supp.)

Ans **BRONCHIAL ASTHMA:** It is characterised by an exaggerated Broncho constrictor response to many stimuli inducing paroxysmal mainly expiratory airflow obstruction, marked dyspnoea and wheezing.

PRECIPITATING FACTORS:
1. Respiratory Infections: bacterial or non bacterial in nature.
2. Allergens: Inhalants like pollens, ingestants like milk, eggs etc.
3. Exercise: especially running.
4. Drugs: like B Blockers.
5. Weather: Sudden changes in the temperature. fog, cold winds.
6. Psychological stress. Ranging from pleasureable excitement in children to stress or worry; or frank endogenous depression.

CLINICAL FEATURES:
1. PREMONITARY SYMPTOMS: Asthmatic aura in the form of sneezing, flatulence, drowsiness or restlessness and irritability are seen. Dry cough may Precede or accompany the attack.
2. PAROXYSMS: They are usually sudden in the middle of night with a sense of oppression in chest going to respiratory distress.

He sits up and leans forward fighting for breath or runs to window to reduce the sense of suffocation.

Wheezing may be heard at a distance with anxiety, cyanosis, perspiration and cold extremities.

O/E: a Tachycardia.
    b. Rales at the base of lungs towards the end of attack.
    c. Plenty of Rhonchi all over.
3. TERMINATION: It either terminates spontaneously or as a result of therapy.
4. DURATION OF ATTACK: It varies from few minutes to several hours.

INVESTIGATIONS:
1. Blood: Shows eosinophillia
2. Sputum Shows the presence of eosinophils and charcot Leyden crystals.

TREATMENT:
I GENERAL:
   1. Avoidance of smoking
   2. Education regarding the disease.
   3. Chest Exercises

II. SPECIFIC TREATMENT:
   1. Hyposensitisation: It is the only specific measure available for prevention of damaging the antigen antibody reaction. It involves the subcutaneous introduction of allergens which are held to be responsible.
   2. In severe cases O_2 inhalation is essential.

STATUS ASTHMATICUS: The usual attack of asthma turns into status Asthmaticus, if bronchodilators are ineffective in relieving the attack after 24 hours or if the attack is so severe that the patient is unable to speak in sentences.

MANAGEMENT:
1. O_2 in high conc.
2. I.V injection of drugs is given
3. 5% glucose saline is given about 100 ml/kg/24 hrs.
4. Correction of Electrolytes. Potassium at the rate of 2meq/100 ml and Sodium Bicarbonate at the rate of 80-100ml of 7.5% solution is given.
5. Use of Bronchodilators.
6. Intubation and assisted ventilation: with endotracheal tube is given.

Q-3. A 40 yrs old smoker has come to you with the complaint of Haemoptysis. Discuss the investigations, Differential diagnosis and give treatment of any one of them. (1975 Supp, 1978, 1978, 1982, 1988 Supp.)

Ans. DIFFERENTIAL DIAGNOSIS :
1. TUBERCULOSIS: The patient complains of evening rise of temperature with cough and Haemoptysis. It is generally associated with decreased appetite and Cachexia. Investigations show Raised E.S.R with positive mantoux test and consolidation in chest X-Ray.
2. PULMONARY INFARCT: It usually starts with pain in chest and Haemoptysis. There is usually a H/O cardiovascular disease. X-Ray shows wedge shaped consolidation.
3. BRONCHOGENIC CA: The patient presents with cough, Haemoptysis, early clubbing with enlarged axillary or cervical lymph nodes. Bronchography is diagnostic.
4. BRONCHITIS: usually in chronic bronchitis the patient brings excessive sputum but with difficulty. On examination the chest movements are slightly restricted with Rhonchi and crepitations at the bases of lungs.
5. MITRAL STENOSIS: It presents with difficulty in respiration with blood stained cough. On examination the first heard sound is loud with opening snap and diastolic murmus in the mitral area.

INVESTIGATIONS:
1. Blood: for TLC, DLC, E.S.R. and blood gas analysis.
2. Mantoux Test.
3. X-Ray chest.
4. Bronchoscopy with lung biopsy.

Treatment of Pul T.B:
1. GENERAL
   a. Rest in bed.
   b. Use of good diet rich in proteins, calories and vitamins.
2. USE OF ANTI TUBERCULAR TREATMENT:
   a. Six month Regimen.
   b. Nine month Regimen.

The drugs like Streptomycin, isoniazid, Rifampicin are used.

Q-4. How would you define chronic Bronchitis? Discuss

in detail its **Complications and management. (1988 Supp.)**

Ans. CHRONIC BRONCHITIS: A patient is said to have C. bronchitis if sputum has been coughed up on most days for at least 3 consecutive months for more than 2 successive years, provided other causes of productive cough such as bronchiectasis and untreated chronic asthma have been excluded.

COMPLICATIONS:

1. RESPIRATORY FAILURE: It is usually recognised from changes in the arterial gas pressure. Type I failure occurs in mild to moderate cases while Type II occurs in patients with several airflow obstruction.
2. PULMONARY HYPERTENSION AND VENTRICULAR FAILURE: The increase in pulmonary artery pressure is due to vasoconstriction and also due to destruction of pulmonary vascular bed. The degree of air flow obstruction, hypoxia, bacterial infection of resptract, oedema of bronchial musosa, oversecretion of bronchial mucus and spasm are liable to precipitate the right ventricular failure.
3. SECONDARY POLYCYTHAEMIA: It is a reflex response of Hypoxaemia.

TREATMENT:

1. GENERAL:
    a. Stop smoking.
    b. Avoidance of dusty and smoke laden atmosphere.
    c. Treatment of any respiratory infection.
2. SPECIFIC
    a. Bronchodilator therapy.
    b. O_2 Therapy: Controlled low concentration O_2 is given
    c. Respiratory Stimulants: are given specially in advanced acidosis.
    d. Mechanical Ventillation: is given in type II Respiratory failure.
    e. Physiotherapy Assisted expectoration is of help in patients who are drowsy because of Co_2 retention.

Q-5. What is Tropical Eosinophilia? Describe it's radiological features.
(1988 Supp.)

Ans. The condition which is more common in the tropics is characterised by an absolute rise of eosinophlic count of 2800/cumm or more in the peripheral blood and associated with respiratory symptoms.

CLINICAL FEATURES:
1. COUGH: In early stages it is dry and hacking later on becomes paroxysmal and is worse at night.
2. DYSPNOEA: There is usually expiratory dyspnoea.
3. FEVER: mild to moderate fever is common with relapses.
4. LOSS OF WEIGHT: Poor appetite with disinclination for evening meal is the predisposing factor.
5. General Weakness and Exhausation.

RADIOLOGICAL FEATURES:
1. Diffuse mottling of lungs usually bilateral and symmetrical.
2. Prominent linear striations radiating from the hilum.
3. Diffuse fan shaped streaks.
4. Ground glass appearance of lung fields.

Q-6. What is Bronchitis? Give its symptoms with Homoeopathic management. (1987.)
Ans. DEFINITION: See Q-4.

SYMPTOMS:
1. COUGH: There is constant or paroxysmal cough which is usually worse during winters or on exposed cold winds or from sudden change of temperature.
2. EXPECTORATION: It is usually variable ranging from little, thin and mucoid to thick, frothy, mucoid and sticky.
3. DIFFICULTY IN RESPIRATION: There is difficulty in breathing when overexerted, while climbing stairs or when taking exercises.

HOMOEOPATHIC MANAGEMENT: See Q-1.

Q-7. A 20 yrs old girl comes to you with Bacterial Pneumonitis. How would you diagnose this condition mention 4 Homoeopathic drugs to treat her condition. (1987 Supp.)

Ans. DIAGNOSIS BY
1. History Taking
2. Sputum Examination.
3. X-Ray chest will show patchy pneumonitis
4. Blood will show: E.S.R, T.L.C, D.L.C. all raised than the normal limits.

1. ARSENIC ALBUM: It is one of the efficient drugs when the fever paroxysm comes at about 12-2 Am/Pm with great weakness and restlessness.

   It is associated with cough with scanty expectoration which is blood stained and offensive smelling. There is increased thirst for small quantities. There is increased sweating with complete loss of appetite.

2. BRYONIA: It is a good Remedy when the onset is insidious with dry short lasting spasmodic cough. It is associated with pain in chest while coughing with increased senstivity to touch and better by lying on the affected side and by pressure.

   There is increased thirst with constipated bowels.

3. SANGUINARIA: It is especially good for (R) sided pneumonitis when there is intense burning in the chest. Cough is usually of gastric origin and is worse by lying on right side.

   Spasmodic cough after influenza. Cough returns with every cold severe soreness in chest and under Right nipple. It is associated with circumscribed redness of cheeks.

4. EUCALYPTUS: It is good for the Pneumonitis of sudden onset following an attack of Influenza. It usually starts with coryza with stuffed up sensation in the nose.

   Fever with foul discharge from all over the body. The cough is productive of thick white offensive mucus. The complaints are usually worse at night.

Q-8. Mention the causes of Asthma. How will you differentiate it from chronic Bronchitis? How will you manage a case of status Asthmaticus? Suggest 3 top

Respiratory System

medicines with their indications. (1980.)

Ans. The causes can be classified into:
1. PRIMARY CAUSES   2. PRECIPITATING CAUSES

The primary can be again discussed under
1. ATOPIC ASTHMA: It is usually due to formation of antibodies IGE against the antigens. Hypersenstivity skin tests are +ve
   It is allergic in origin
2. NON ATOPIC: No allergic causes are seen to be responsible. But it is due to intrinsic mechanism of the Immune System of body.

PRECIPITATING CAUSES: See Q-2.

BRONCHIAL ASTHMA	CHRONIC BRONCHITIS
1. DEFINITION: A syndrome Characterised by increased responsiveness of trachea and Bronchi to various stimuli	Chronic Inflammation of mucus membrane of trachea and bronchi is called Bronchitis.
2. ETIOLOGY: Hypersenstivity of the individual to specific allergens.	Infections, smoking in combination are responsible.
3. Family H/O allergy is generally seen.	Not seen
4. Dyspnoea is very marked.	cough with dyspnoea is marked.
5. ON AUSCULTATION: Wheeze and Rhonchi are heard all over the chest.	Rhonchi with crepitations are heard at the lung bases.
6. X-RAY CHEST: is normal	It shows increased Broncho vesicular markings.
7. Constitutional Symptoms are very marked.	They are not significant.
8. Blood Examination shows Eosinophilla with raised levels of IGE.	It is normal.

MANAGEMENT OF STATUS AS THMATICUS: See Q-2.

1. ARSENIC ALBUM: See Q-7.

2. PSORINUM: It is useful when there is a history of suppressed skin eruptions or an evidence of latent psora.

Asthma with dyspnoea which is aggravated when sitting but better by lying down and keeping the arms spread

wide apart. Dry hard cough with great weakness in chest. Feeling of ulceration under the chest with pain better by lying down. Cough returns every winter from suppressed eruptions.
3. IPECAC: It is suited to those persons who are feeble and catch cold easily. There is dyspnoea with constriction in chest.

Yearly attacks of difficult shortness of breathing. Cough incessant and violent with every breath. Chest seems full of phlegm but nothing comes out. It is good when constant nausea with clean tongue is associated with it.

All the complaints are worse from lying down in a warm moist room.

Q-9. Describe the causes and clinical features of pleurisy with effusion. Indicate 4 Homoeopathic drugs. (1985.)
Ans. CAUSES:
1. Infection: T.B, Pneumonia, Fungal Infections,
2. Congestive causes: C.C.F, Constrictive pericarditis.
3. malignancy: Bronchogenic CA, malignant neoplasms of stomach, Lymphomas.
4. Thrombosis of azygous vein.
5. Trauma and penetrating wounds of chest
    a. Bronchopleural fistula
    b. Subphrenic abscess.
6. Systemic Infections.
    a. S.L.E
    b. R.A
    C. Infectious mononueleosis.

SYMPTOMS:
1. ONSET is acute with attack of pleuritic pain.
2. DYSPNOEA: It usually depends on the rate of collection and amount of fluid.
3. Dry cough with marked constitutional Symptoms.
4. Loss of weight with fever.

SIGNS
1. ON INSPECTION
    a. Patient is seen lying on the affected side.
    b. Diminished mobility of chest on affected side.

2. ON PALPATION
   a. Trachea is shifted to the opposite side.
   b. Diminished vocal fremitus.
3. ON PERCUSSION
   a. Stony dullness
   b. Skodiac Resonance above the level of fluid.
4. ON AUSCULTATION
   a. Breath Sounds are diminished or absent
   b. Bronchial Breathing in early stages.
   c. Diminished or absent vocal Resonance.
   d. Rales may be heard at the base of the opposite lung due to congestion.

HOMOEOPATHIC DRUGS:

1. KALI CARB: It is good for (R) sided affections when there are sharp stitching pains which constantly go right through the back. The patient is unable to lie on the affected side. The complaints are worse early morning around 3 A M.

Whole chest is very sensitive. All symptoms are better by leaning forward.

2. APIS: The respiration is difficult with a constant Hurried breathing. Feels as if he could not draw another breath. The pains are of burning nature which are worse at 3 A.M/P.M with swelling of lower lids.
3. BRYONIA: See Q-7.
4. ARS ALBUM: See Q-7.

Q-10. Describe the clinical features of lobar Pneumonia. What are the indications of 4 Homoeopathic drugs. (1977, 1978 Supp, 1981, 1983, 1984.)

Ans.   **ETIOLOGY:**

1. BACTERIAL: Pneumococus, staphylococi, Haemophilus influenzae
2. VIRAL: Small pox virus, Resp synctical virus
3. RICKETISSAE: Coxiella Burnetti Pneumoniae.
4. MY COPLASMA: mycoplasma prevmonal, steven Johanson Syndrome.
5. PROTOZOAL: Entamoeba Histoly tica.
6. PREDISPOSING CAUSES

a. Factors which reduces the general resistance of individual like; old age, uncontrolled diabetes
  b. Viral Infections of upper respiratory Tract
  c. Chronic Respiratory Diseases.
  d. Alcohlism

SYMPTOMS:
1. General Constitutional symptoms: like malaise, fever, chills with rigors and vomiting are seen.
2. PULMONARY SYMPTOMS: of cough, dyspnoea and rusty sputum raised with difficulty.
3. FEVER: Onset is sudden with chills and rises to 39-40°C
4. Pleural symptoms: Pain in chest worse by cough, deep breathing or movement usually localised to the site of inflammation.

SIGNS
1. Slight impairment of percussion note over the affected area with diminished breath sounds.
2. Signs of consolidation.
   a. Reduced movement on affected side
   b. Increased vocal Fremitus.
   c. Raised vocal Resonance
3. Signs of Resolution.
   a. Rales and impaired resonance over the affected area.

HOMOEOPATHIC DRUGS:
1. BRYONIA: See Q-7.
2. BALSAM PERU: See Q-1.
3. EUCALYPTUS: See Q-7.
4. IPECAC: See Q-8.

Q-11. What is pneumothorax? What are its types. Describe the features of Acute Pneumothorax. (1982)

Ans. Presence of air in the pleural space making an air containing pleural cavity, is Pneumothorax.

TYPES OF PNEUMOTHORAX:
1. CLOSED: The communication between the Pleura and lungs seals off as the lung deflates and does not reopen.

Respiratory System

The air is gradually absorbed and the lung re expands.
2. OPEN: The communication is generally with a bronchus and does not seal off when the lung collapses. The pressure of air in the pleural space becomes equal to the atmospheric pressure.
3. TENSION: The communication between the pleura and lungs persists but is small and acts as a one way valve which allows the air to enter the pleural space during inspiration and coughing but prevents it from escaping.

It causes compression of the underlying lung with mediastinal displacement on the opposite side.

FEATURES OF ACUTE PNEUMOTHORAX:
1. Onset is sudden with pain or feeling of tightness in the chest on affected side.
2. The pains are aggravated by deep breathing.
3. There is increasing dyspnoea with cyanosis.
4. The patient gives a TOXIC LOOK.

Q-12. Discuss the etiology, pathology and clinical features of COAD. Name 3 important Homoeopathic drugs (1991)

Ans. **ETIOLOGY:**
1. INFECTIONS: a. As a result of acute Bronchitis.
b. Infective focus in upper respiratory tract, nasal sinuses or tonsils.
2. SMOKING: particularly of cigaretes.
3. AIR POLLUTION: due to industrial fumes and dust.
4. GENERAL ILLNESS: Which favours infection like obesity, alcohlism, chronic renal diseases.

PATHOLOGY: There is hypertrophy of mucus secreting glands with an increase in the number of goblet cells in the bronchi and bronchioles with a decrease in the cilliated cells.

Mucosal oedema and permanent structural damage of the airways causes the reduction in the calibre of air passages. Air is trapped in the alveoli because the degree of obstruction is greater during expiration.

Ultimately over distension of the alveoli results and

disruption of their walls may ocur leading to emphysema.
For rest See Q-4, Q-6.

Q-13. Discuss the Differential Diagnosis of a case of chronic cough. (Supp 1991.)

Ans. The causes can be grouped under 3 categories
1. Inflammatory causes including infections.
2. Mechanical or Irritating causes
3. Reflex causes

CAUSES	PRESENTATION
A. UPPER RESPIRATORY INFECTIONS	
1. Tonsillitis	A tendency for the throat to be affected on either exposure to cold or from taking cold things. It is associated with irritation and pain in throat. O/E tonsils are enlarged and Congested.
2. Pharyngitis	Hawking cough is diagnostic with painful swallowing < when empty swallowing O/E. Pharynx appears to be congested.
3. Laryngitis	Hawking cough with voice changes, of ten chronic in nature must hawk and clear the throat constantly to get the voice clear.
4. Tracheitis	Hawking cough seen specially in cigarete smokers. There is soreness behind the upper sternum.
5. Chronic sinusitis	It is seen in chronic maxillary sinusitis. O/E Tenderness of sinuses with post nasal dripping and obstruction of nose.
B. LOWER RESP. TRACT	
6. Chronic Bronchitis	Wheezing cough associated with expectoration. Irritants like dusts, pollen, gases are responsible. O/A: B/L Rhonchi are heard at the lung bases with prolonged expiration and expiratory wheeze.

CAUSES	PRESENTATION
7. T.B.	a. Irritable dry cough < in the early morning and on going to bed. b. With Haemoptysis, low grade fever and Nocturnal sweats.
8. Tropical Eosinophillia	Dry tickling cough which is paroxysmal at night with expiratory dyspnoea. It is associated with marked constitutional Symptoms and an absolute increase in the EOSINOPHILIC COUNT.
9. Bronchogenic CA	Cough usually with mucopurulent sputum, haemoptysis and failure of chest infections to resolve. Weakness, loss of weight anorexia and fever are associated. X-Ray shows signs of collapse
10. COAD	Chronic productive cough with signs of emphysematous chest.
11. Bronchiectasis	Cough with copious purulent expectoration clubbing of fingers and signs of Toxaemia.

C. MECHANICAL/IRRITATING CAUSES
1. Upper Respiratory Tract
   a. Enlarged Tonsils
   b. Elongated uvvla
   c. Smoker's Throat
2. MEDIASTINAL CAUSES
   a. Aortic Aneurysm
   b. Enlarged mediastinal glands.
   c. Growth of Thymus
   d. Pericardial Effusion
   e. Dilated (L) Atrium in mitral Stenosis

D. REFLEX CAUSES
1. Diseases of Ext ear.
2. Overloading of stomach
3. Distension of colon

CAUSES	PRESENTATION
E. PSYCHOGENIC CAUSES	
Hysterical cough	Common in females No organic lesion is found
F. ENVIRONMENTAL OCCUPATIONAL CAUSES	H/O occupational exposure
a. Pneumoconiosis	X-Ray shows diffuse fibrosing changes in both lungs symmetrically.
b. Sarcoidosis	
c. Asbestosis	
d. Sillicosis.	

Q-14. Mention various causes where chest is Hyper-Resonant on percussion. Describe the clinical features and complications of a case of Emphysema of Lungs (1982 Supp.)

Ans. **CAUSES OF HYPERRESONANT CHEST:**
1. Emphysema
2. Pneumothorax
3. An area above the pleural effusion in SKODIAC RESONANCE.

CLINICAL FEATURES:
For symptoms See Q-4.

SIGNS: The important signs are
A. **ON INSPECTION**
1. Chest is Barrel Shaped
2. The chest movements are diminished.
3. Fullness of supra clavicular Fossa.
4. Patient is seen in the posture of leaning forward with pursed lips often cyanosed.
5. Raised JVP.

B. **ON PALPATION**
1. V.F is diminished
2. A reduction in the length of trachea palpable above the sternal notch.
3. The chest expansion is diminished on palpation

C. **ON PERCUSSION.** There is Hyper resonant sound on percussion.
D. **ON AUSCULTATION**
1. Breath sounds are diminished or absent, with proolonged expiration.

For complications See Q-6.

Q-15. A young man has come to you with a History of cough, fever and weight loss for sometime. How will you investigate such a case? Give your diagnosis with 4 Homoeopathic medicines. (1979, 1982 Supp.)

Ans. Clinically it is can be diagnosed as a case of PULMONARY T.B.
The investigations are:
1. Sputum for A.F.B.
2. Blood: TLC, DLC, E.S.R.
3. mantoux test.
4. X-Ray chest.

HOMOEOPATHIC MEDICINES:
1. Sanguinaria: See Q-7.
2. Bacllinum: See Q-1.
3. Arsenic Album: See Q-7
4. Psorinum See Q-8.

Q-16. What are the common causes of dullness on percussion of chest? How will you differentiate Lobar pneumonia from plural effusion? (1976, 1983)

Ans. **CAUSES OF DULLNESS ON PERCUSSION:**
1. Pleural Effusion
2. Pneumonia
3. Thickened pleura
4. T.B of Lung
5. Fibrosis Lung
6. Collapse of Lung
7. Atelectasis.

	LOBAR PNEUMONIA	**PLEURAL EFFUSION**
1.	DEFINITION: It is a patchy consolidation involving a lobe of lung.	The collection of fluid in the pleural cavity is plural effusion.

	LOBAR PNEUMONIA	PLEURAL EFFUSION
2.	ETIOLOGY: Usually bacterial in origin	It can be due to a. Bacteria b. Tumours c. Congestion
3.	SKODIAC RESONANCE is absent	is characteristic of Pleural effusion.
4.	CONSTITUTIONAL SYMPTOMS are very marked.	They are less markedly seen.
5.	AGE AND SEX: It occurs in old and debilitated persons with equal sex incidence.	It is seen usually in young and middle aged subjects but can be seen in any age group.
6.	ONSET: is acute.	It is generally insidious
7.	Rusty sputum is raised.	Here the cough is dry
8.	Impaired note on percussion.	It is completly flat note.
9.	No displacement of mediastinum.	It is displaced to the opposite side.
10.	Breath sounds are bronchal type, if massive then they are absent.	They are completely absent.

Q-17. Write short notes on
1. **PNEUMOCONIOSIS:** (1988 Supp)

It refers to the group of diseases caused by mineral dusts. The dust particles after inhalation are conveyed by macrophages from the Bronchial mucosa to minute foci of lymphoid tissue throughout the lungs.

The coal workers pneumo coniosis can be of 2 types:

1. SIMPLE COAL WORKER'S PNEUMOCONIOSIS: It does not progress further if the miner leaves the industry

2. PROGRESSIVE MASSIVE FIBROSIS: In this form larger dense masses single or multiple occur mainly in the upper lobes. These may be irregular in shape and may cavitate. Tuberculosis acts as a complication of the progression of disease.

CLINICAL FEATURES:
1. Cough and sputum from associated Bronchitis.
2. The sputum is black and foul smelling.
3. Breathlessness on exertion.
4. CAPLAN'S SYNDROME: When R.A is associated with fibrotic nodules in the peripheral lung fields it is called caplan's Syndrome.

2. **BRONCHOSCOPY** (1988 SUPP.)

The method of examining the lower respiratory tract with the help of a FIBROPTIC BRONCHOSCOPE is called BRONCHOSCOPY.

METHOD: The flexible fibroptic bronchoscope is introduced into the tracheobronchial tree via the nose, mouth, tracheostomy or endotracheal tube permitting inspection of trachea and all segmental bronhioles and orfices.

The nasopharynx and oropharyngolarynx are similarly examined at the same time.

Abnormal lesions are brushed or biopsed and specimens are sent for histological, cytological and pathological investigations.

IMPORTANCE:
1. It evaluates the cause of Haemoptysis.
2. It aids in localisation of airway obstruction.
3. Helps in the removal of tenacious secretions and mucus plugs.
4. Helpful in the treatment of ATELECTASIS.
5. Helps in the removal of foreign body.
6. It is beneficial in Lung lavage.

3. **COMMON COLD AND HOMOEOPATHIC REMEDIES** (1987, 1988 SUPP.)

It is also called coryza.

ETIOLOGY:
Although a definite cause is not known but few microorganisms are held to be responsible
1. Bacterias:
2. Viruses:
3. Lowered Resistance of the person.

CLINICAL FEATURES:
1. Onset is sudden with a burning and tickling sensation in the nose with sneezing.

2. The throat feels dry, sore with fullness of head and profuse watery nasal discharge.

COMPLICATIONS:
1. Chronic Sinusitis
2. Eustachian Catarrh.
3. Otitis Media.

HOMOEOPATHIC MEDICINES:
1. Allium cepa   4. Influenzinum.
2. Euphrasia
3. Rhustox

4. **ACUTE SINUSITIS AND ITS MANAGEMENT** (1987 Supp.)

The inflammation of the mucus membrane lining the paranasal sinuses is called SINUSITIS.

ETIOLOGY:
1. It is the extension from acute Rhinitis
2. Dental infection like apical abscess, oro antral fistula
3. The bacterias like staphylococcus, Streptococci, pneumococci are responsible.

SYMPTOMS:
1. CONSTITUTIONAL SYMPTOMS: They consist of fever, malaise, lack of appetite and body aches.
2. NASAL OBSTRUCTION: Which can be unilateral or bilateral.
3. Pain in the sinuses with discharge of thick, yellow, green discharge on blowing the nose.
4. Catarrhal Headache in frontals. It is severe in forenoon and vanes off by mid day.
5. The sense of smell is diminished but sometimes altered sense of smell is also seen.
6. O/E: The sinuses are tender on palpation.

MANAGEMENT:
1. Use of nasal decongestants.
2. Steam inhalation.
3. Homoeopathic drugs like Nux vomica, Amm Carb, Kali Bichromicum can be used.

5. **PNEUMO THORAX:** What is the need of Artifical Pneumothorax:(1986)

See Q-11

NEED FOR ARTIFICAL PNEUMO THORAX: It was an old techinique being followed in the treatment of Pulmonary T.B and also in several chest operations and in mediastinal operations.

But it is completely obsolete now.

6. **PULMONARY OEDEMA;** (1985)

The term pulmonary oedema may be regarded as an increase in the fluid content of the extravascular tissues of the lung.

CAUSES:
1. CARDIAC ORIGIN
   a. L.V failure
   b. myocardial Infarction
   c. mitral stenosis
2. NON CARDIAC ORIGIN
   a. Excessive fluid intake.
   b. Shock
   c. Inhalation of noxious fumes and gases.
   d. Aspiration of contents in Pleural cavity

CLINICAL PRESENTATION
1. Onset is sudden with oppression in the chest and dyspnoea.
2. Cough: Patient constantly coughs and brings up frothy sputum.
3. Feeble pulse with sweating and fall of temperature.
4. X-Ray shows Bats wing appearance.

7. **HAEMOPTYSIS** (1974 SUPP, 1984, 1985) See Q-3

8. **SKODIAC RESONANCE:** (1974 Supp, 1985)

A clear high pitched note occuring above the level of pleural effusion i,e over the lung that is relaxed but still containing air.

It is usually seen in Pleural effusion.

9. **BRONCHIAL BREATH SOUNDS:** (1984)

They are usually a type in which there is a definite pause between inspiration and expiration.
It has the following features:
1. Both phases are harsh in character with a distinct pause.

2. They may be heard normally over the trachea.
3. They are heard in T.B. and Bronchopneumonia. Close to the tumour, to a large bronchus, lung collapse, infarction.
4. In empyema specially in children it is often present.

VARIANTS OF BRONCHIAL BREATH SOUNDS
1. Tubular Breathing   3. Amphoric Breathing.
2. Cavernous Breathing

10. **CHEYNE STOKE'S BREATHING:** (1981, 1983)

It consists of rythmical waxing and waning of respirations ie alternations of Hyperpnoea and Apnoea.

Anything that causes Anoxaemia of the Respiratory centre results in Cheyne Stoke's Breathing.

MECHANISM: Apnoea results in the accumalation of CO_2 in the body thereby reawakening the centre of respiration and causes Hyperventilation which in turn removes the excess of CO_2 whereupon the centre goes to sleep again.

CAUSES:
1. LESIONS OF BRAIN:
    a. Meningitis
    b. Cerbral abscess
    c. Cerebral Haemorrhage
2. CARDIAC CAUSES
    a. Left ventricular failure
    b. Hypertension due to Renal Diseases
3. POISONS AND TOXINS
    a. Opium and Barbiturates
    b. Uraemia.

11. **CLUBBING** (1983.)

The drum stick appearance of fingers with the obliteration of angle between the nail bed and it's base is called CLUBBING.

CAUSES
1. RESPIRATORY CAUSES
    a. CA of Bronchus
    b. Bronchiectasis
    c. Lung abscess
    d. COAD

2. CARDIAC CAUSES
   a. Congenital cyanotic diseases   b. SABE
3. GASTRO INTESTINAL CAUSES
   a. Cirrhosis
   b. Ulcerative colitis
4. ENDOCRINE CAUSES
   a. myxoedema.

STAGES OF CLUBBING:
1. STAGE - I Thickening of nail bed with increased circulation.
2. STAGE II Gradual obliteration of the angle between the nail bed and base of nail.
3. STAGE III Longitudinal and Horizontal furrowing.
4. STAGE IV Thickened phalanges with a typical appearance of DRUMSTICK.

12. **RHONCHI** (1982.)

They are the adventitious sounds in the respiratory tract due to spasm of bronchial wall because of
a. Swelling or oedema.
b. Spasm
c. Collection of secretions.

They are usually indicative of BRONCHOSPASM. They are usually found in Bronchitis, Asthma and Pneumonia or in any spasmodic affections of the bronchus.

13. **EPISTAXIS:** (1982)

Bleeding from the nose is called epistaxis.

CAUSES:
1. INJURY: blows, fracture, foreign body.
2. INFECTIONS: Diptheria, Influenza, Scarlet fever.
3. NEW GROWTHS: Adenoids, polypi, malignancy.
4. ULCERATION: Syphilis, T.B, leprosy
5. GENERAL CAUSES: Hypertension.
6. SEVERE GENERALISED INFECTIONS: measles, small pox.
7. IDIOPATHIC:

TREATMENT:
1. Application of cold sponges
2. Use of adrenaline

3. Plugging of nose with bandage.
4. Drugs like Amm Carb, millefolium, Lachesis can be used.

14. COMPARE BRONCHIECTASIS AND LUNG ABSCESS (1989, 1991)

	BRONCHIECTASIS	LUNG ABSCESS.
1.	DEFINITION: It is abnormal dilatation of Bronchioles	It is a form of lung tissue consolidation in which there is destruction of lung parenchyma.
2.	ETIOLOGY: a. congenital	Bacterial infection of a pulmonary infarct or of a Collapsed lung may produce it.
b.	Primary T.B	
c.	Suppurative pneumonia.	
3.	CLINICAL FEATURES	
a.	Chronic cough usually productive of excessive sputum by postural changes.	It is comparitively less.
b.	Constitutinal symptoms absent.	They are well marked.
4.	PERCUSSION NOTE. may be slightly impaired.	It is dull on percussion.
5.	Signs are usually confined to both the lung bases.	They are be seen anywhere either in upper middle or lower zone.
6.	O/A: Crepitations are over the chest particularly in bases.	Crepitations in middle zone with ocasional Rhonchi.
7.	RADIOLOGICAL EXAMINATION shows dilatation of bronchi with destruction.	Patchy consolidation is seen.
8.	PROGNOSIS: is generally poor.	It is good if controlled in time.
9.	TREATMENT:	
a.	Postural drainage	Use of antibiotics.
b.	use of chemo therapy	
10.	SURGICAL ROLE: is definite.	It is not unless complications set in.

Respiratory System

15. **TEITZ SYNDROME** (1989.)
It is a form of costochondritis which affects particularly the 2nd and 3rd COSTAL CARTILAGE.

ETIOLOGY:
1. Bacterias like staphylococcus, pneumococci.
2. Viral Infections

CLINICAL FEATURES:
1. Pain and swelling of the chest wall, in costal cartilages
2. Fever with constitutional symptoms.
3. O/P; There is tenderness on palpation.

TREATMENT:
1. Use of Antibiotics.
2. Use of analgesics.
3. Drugs like Pix Liquida, Ran Bulbosus, Rhus tox can be used.

16. **SMOKING:** (1991) It is one of the commonest social problem in young and old sex of society.

The young males adopt smoking as a result of following factors:
1. To be relieved from sufferings and tensions of life
2. To accompany the Friend circle.
3. To show off the dominancy of adolescents.

DANGERS OF SMOKING:
1. Chronic Lung infections.
2. Bronchogenic CA.
3. Coronary Artery Disease.

TO GET RID OF THE HABIT OF SMOKING: following Homoeopathic drugs can be used.
1. Tabacum
2. Avena Sativa
3. Sulphuric acid.

17. **PLEURAL RUB** (1978.)

These sounds are due to rubbing of the 2 surfaces of pleura in early pleurisy. They ocur when the two inflamed surfaces rub against each other during inspiration as well as during the corresponding period of expiration.

They remain unchanged on coughing and are intenstified by the pressure of stethoscope. They are best heard where areas of pleurisy are more frequent i.e. in axillae and beneath the nipples.

18. **TUBULAR BREATHING:** (1982)

It is one of the variants of Bronchial breathing. It is high pitched breathing with a small but distinct pause and with inspiration equal to expiration.

HEARD IN: Lobar and Broncopneumonia.

19. **COR PULMONALE** (1977, 1983.)

The disease of heart resulting from lung diseases is called COR PÚLMONALE.

CLASSIFICATION:
1. ACUTE: Acute pulmonary enbolism
2. CHRONIC:
    a. COAD
    b. Inflammatory Lung Diseases like T.B, Bronchiectasis
    c. Pulmonary vessel Diseases: Recurrent pul enbolism, Polyarteritis Nodosa.

20. **EMPYEMA** (1981)

The collection of pus in the pleural cavity is called EMPYEMA.

ETIOLOGY:
1. Extension from lung infection Pneumonia, Lung abscess.
2. Secondary to Suppuration in adjacent structures: like T.B. of Rib, paravertebral abscess.
3. Penetrating wounds of chest.
4. Subphrenic abscess.

SYMPTOMS:
1. THOSE OF PRIMARY DISEASE: Imperfect recovery in pneumonia cases or sudden increase in fevers.
2. THOSE DUE TO MECHANICAL EFFECTS: chest pain, cough with sputum, dyspnoea.
3. DUE TO TOXAEMIA: malaise, anorexia, sweats, loss of weight with clubbing.

SIGNS: See pleural effusion

TREATMENT:
1. Aspiration of pus under water seal drainage
2. Use of Antibiotics:

21. **HARRISON'S SULCUS:** (1981)

It is a transverse groove passing outwards from Xiphisternum as far as mid axillary line sometimes occuring along the line of diaphragmatic attachment. It is associated with a PIGEON CHEST OR RACHITIC CHEST.

22. **HAEMOPHILUS INFLUENZAE :** 1992

It is a bacteria which exists in cocco bacillary form in Cultures but shows bacillary morphology in C.S.F. of patients with meningitis.

It is nearly aerobic but can also grow anaerobically. Culture yields Capsulated and non Capsulatea Colonies. The Capsulated forms are more Virulent.

The organsins have been classified into 6 types designated a to B is responsible for most of the serious infections.

Around 60-80% of children below 3 yrs harbour the organism in the upper respiratory tract.

It Causes the following Lesions.

1. Hamophilus influenzae meningitis
2. Secondary Infection causes broncho Pneumonia and Suppurative pulmonary lesions..

It is treated by Antibiotics

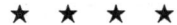

11. HAEMOPOETIC SYSTEM

**Q-1. What is Haemolytic anaemia? Discuss the causes, laboratory investigations with management.
(1987 supp. 1988.)**

Ans. Normal life span of R.B.C. is 120 days. Old cells are removed from the circulation mildly deformed cells are phagocytosed in the spleen and grossly damaged cells are destroyed in the circulation itself. When the lifespan of R.B.C. falls below 120 days Haemolysis becomes excessive and Anaemia is likely to develop.

ETIOLGOY:
The causes of Haemolysis are:
1. A decrease in the surface area or volume ratio of cells: Hereditary spherocytosis, autoimmune Haemolytic anaemia, drug induced haemolysis.
2. Defect in the structure of the R.B.C membrane e.g. Paroxysmal Nocturnal Haemoglobinuria and drug induced haemolysis.
3. Increased Internal viscosity: eg. sickle cell anaemia, Heinz body Haemolytic anaemia.
4. Hypersplenism.

LABORATORY INVESTIGATIONS.
1. Tests to detect the presence of Haemolysis: Although the method is to know the life span but it is not easily available everywhere thereby following can be used.
(1) Total Reticulocyte count.
(a) Serum Billirubin.
(b) Reduction of S. Haptoglobin
(c) Increase in S. Lactic Dehydrogenase.
2. Blood Film Examination under the microscope
3. Demonstration of Antibodies by COOMBS TEST.

4. Osmotic Fragility Test
5. Sucrose Haemolysis and Ham's acid serum Test are diagnostic.

MANAGEMENT:
1. Transfusion of packed Red cells.
2. In acute Intravascular Haemolysis emergency transfusion is needed to avoid cardiorespiratory failure.
3. Folic acid supplements are given.
4. Administration of corticosteroids and immuno depressants.
5. Splenectomy is done.

Q-2. What is meagloblastic anaemia? Give its causes and treatment. (1988 Supp.)

Ans. Anaemia resulting from deficiency of vit B_{12} and Folic acid is called meagloblastic Anaemia.

ETIOLOGY
A. DEFICIENCY OF VIT B12
1. Inadequate Intake:
   a. Strict vegetarians.
   b. Extremely poor diet.
2. Malabsorption
   a. Pernicious Anaemia.
   b. Gastrectomy.
   c. Intestinal Stagnant loop Syndrome.
   d. Chrons Disease.
   e. malabsorption Syndrome.
B. DEFICIENCY OF FOLIC ACID
   a. In adequate Intake.
   b. malabsorption Due to Tropical Sprue, malabsorption Syndrome.
   c. Excessive Demands - Pregnancy, lactation, chronic Haemolytic anaemias.
   d. Drugs like Antiepileptics.
   e. Metabolic: Homocystinuria.
C. DEFECTIVE DNA SYNTHESIS
   a. use of cytotoxic drugs.
   b. In born errors of metabolism.

TREATMENT:

1. In vit B12 Deficiency: Initially Hydroxy cobal amine 1000 mcg Im injections are given for 2-3 weeks.
2. The patient is kept on the maintainence dose of 500-900 mcg in every 3 months for life.
3. In folate Deficiency: Initially 5mg of Folic acid is given orally for at least 4 months.
4. Blood Transfusion of packed cells is given in cases of anaemia CRISIS.
5. Treatment of any Infection.
6. Use of Iron Therapy: by mouth is also essential.
7. Packed platelats are given if purpura or Haemorrhages occur.

Q-3. Mention various causes of Generalised Lympha denopathy. Mention 4 important causes of investigations and treatment of any one of them. (1988 Supp)

Ans. CAUSES OF GENERALISED LYMPHADENOPATHY:
1. Tubercular Lymphadenitis.
2. Syphilitic Lymphadenopathy
3. malignant Lymphadenopathy
4. Infectious mononucleosis.

INVESTIGATIONS REQUIRED.
1. mantoux test.
2. V.D.R.L. test for syphilis.
3. Blood test for the presence of specific antibodies.
4. Paul bunnel test for I.M.
5. X-Ray chest and ultrasound of abdomen to locate the site of malignancy.

TREATMENT OF TUBERCULAR LYMPHADENOPATHY:
See Q-3 of Respiratory System.

Q-4. What is iron deficiency Anaemia? Give its causes, and complications with 3 Homoeopathic drugs. Explain in brief the metabolism of Iron. (1977, 1982, 1987, 1991 Supp.)

Ans. The anaemia resulting from the nutritional deficiency of iron is called IRON DEFICIENCY ANAEMIA.

CAUSES:
I   INCREASED PHYSIOLOGICAL REQUIREMENT:
   1. Rapid growth spurt in adolescents.
   2. menstruating females
   3. Pregnancy
II PATHOLOGICAL BLOOD LOSS
   1. menorrhagia
   2. Bleeding from G.I.T in the form of Bleeding piles P.U.S, intestinal infestations.
   3. From urinary Tract: Recurrent Haematuria, Haemoglobinuria.
   4. Regular Blood Donation
   5. Hereditary Haemorrhagic Telengectasia.
III NUTRITIONAL DEFECTS.
   1. Low Iron Diet: Pure Vegetarians.
   2. Poverty
   3. Presence of inhibitors in diet
IV POOR ABSORPTION OF IRON
   1. Achlorhydria
   2. Gastrectomy
V   EXCESS IRON LOSS
   1. Marked Exfoliation seen in psoriasis.
   2. After git infection
   3. Intravascular Haemolysis.

COMPLICATIONS:
1. Plummer Vinson Syndrome
2. C.C.F
3. Papilloedema with raised intracranial tension
4. Alopecia
5. menorrhagia

HOMOEOPATHIC DRUGS:
1. FERRUM METALLICUM: It is best suited to young weakly persons who are anaemic and chlorotic with pseudo plethora who flush easily with oversensitiveness. They are aggravated after any active effort.

Pallor of skin, mucus membranes with alternate redness. There is voracious appetite with vomiting in mouthful. All the complaints are better by slow motion.

2. **ARS ALBUM:** It is suited to the persons of lax and flabby musculature with the complaints resulting from loss of vital fluids.

All the complaints have a marked PERIODICITY. There is great anguish with restlessness.

Face is pale, swollen cachectic and yellow covered with sweat. There is circumcribed flushing of cheeks.

3. **CHINA:** It is a good remedy for anaemia resulting from loss of vital fluids together with nervous erethism. It is usually suited to chronic cases. Face is always bloated with red and sometimes sallow complexion.

The pains are severe which are aggravated from slightest touch but better by hard pressure.

METABOLISM OF IRON: Iron from the food is absorbed from the upper small intestines mainly in the ferrous form bound to amino acids and sugars.

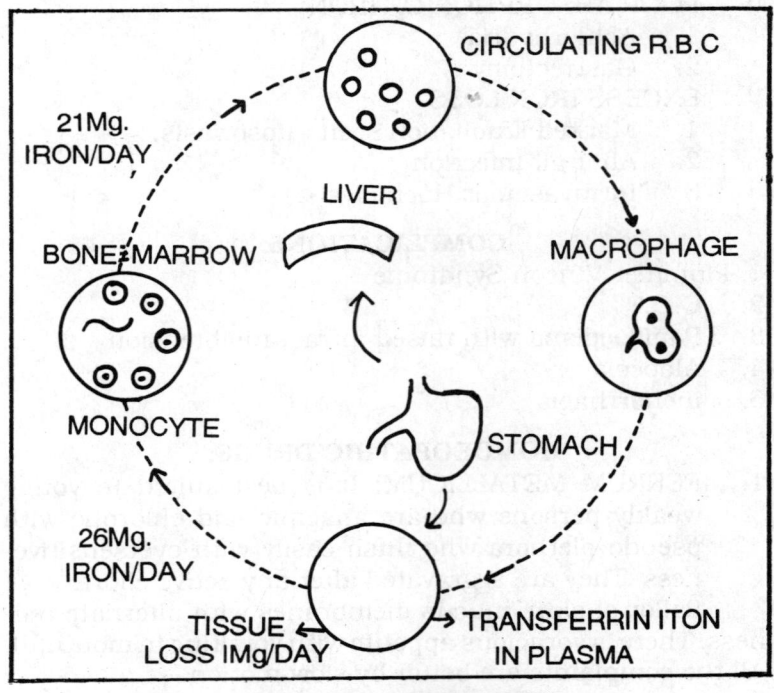

(METABOLISM OF IRON)

Haemopoetic System

Iron readily takes the inabsorbable Ferric form but the low Ph of stomach contents help to preserve it in the Ferrous form.

Iron reaches the cells by IRON TRANSPORT SYSTEM OF TRANSFERRIN. Iron for erythropoesis comes mainly from transferrin and almost all iron absorbed from the gut goes to the bone marrow to be used by the developing red cells.

Q-5. What is pernicious anaemia? Give the causes and clinical features with Homoeopathic Treatment. (1986)

Ans. PERNICIOUS ANAEMIA: The anaemia resulting from the deficiency of Intrinsic factor is called pernicious anaemia.

ETIOLOGY.
1. Lack of Intrinsic factor
2. Auto immune disease.
3. Genetic factor is predominantly important.

SYMPTOMS:
1. Weakness, pallor, lassitude, tingling sensation, palpitation due to anaemia.
2. Recurrent diarrhoea and abdominal pain.
3. Soreness of tongue
4. Neurological symptoms due to subacute combined Degeneration of spinal cord.
5. Fever.

SIGNS
1. Pallor and lemon Yellow discolouration of the skin
2. Red, raw and bald tongue as a result of glossitis.
3. Cardiac dilatation with the haemic murmur.
4. Pins and needle sensation in fingers and toes.
5. Features of involvement of posterior and lateral column of spinal cord due to axonal degeneration and demyelination may develop.
6. Mental disturbances may be present.
7. Spleen is palpable rarely

HOMOEOPATHIC TREATMENT: See Q-4.

Q-6. Describe Hodgkin's Disease. How will you treat it. Suggest 3 drugs with their characteristics. Give the classification and staging of disease. (1982. 1982 Supp 1985, 1986, 1989, 1992.)

Ans. HODGKIN'S DISEASE: The malignant disease of lymphoid cells is called Hodgkin's disease.

CLASSIFICATION OF LYMPHOMAS
1. Hodgkin's Type
2. Non Hodgkin's.

CLINICAL FEATURES:
1. Onset: is insidious with enlargement of one group of superficial nodes which usually fluctuate in size.
2. The nodes are involved in the following order a cervical b. axillary c. Internal mammary glands d. Intra abdominal.
3. The nodes are discrete with rubbery consistency and painless.
4. Splenomeagly is also seen.
5. Pressure symptoms like dysphagia, dyspnoea, venous obstruction, jaundice and paraplegia may occur.
6. Constitutional Symptoms include anorexia with loss of weight, progressive weakness and drenching night sweats.
5. Classical fever of PEL EBSTEIN is present.
6. Pruritus is also seen.

STAGING:
Stage I   Involvement of a single lymph node region or extralymphatic site (IE)

Stage II   Involvement of 2 or more lymph node regions or an extra lymphatic site and lymph node regions on the same side above or below the diaphragm. (IIE)

Stage III   Involvement of lymph nodes regions on both sides of the diaphragm with (IIIE) or without (III) localised extra lymphatic involvement or involvement of the spleen (IIIS) or both (IIISE)

Stage IV   Diffuse involvement of one or more extra lymphatic tissues like liver or bone marrow.

Haemopoetic System

TREATMENT:
1. Radiotherapy: It is given for a period of 4 weeks
2. Chemotherapy.
3. Combined chemo and Radio therapy.

HOMOEOPATHIC DRUGS:
1. IODUM: See Q-10 of Endocrine.
2. CALC IOD: See Q-10 of Endocrine System
3. CALC CARB: See Q-11 of Endocrine System.

Q-7. What is Leukaemia? Give the types, clinical features of chronic myeloid Leukaemia. (1977, 1982.)

Ans. LEUKAEMIA: They are a group of neoplastic disorders affecting mainly the leucopoetic tissues in the body and characterised by the presence of leucocytosis, immature leucocytes in the peripheral blood.

The proliferation of these immature cells in the bone marrow resulting in the suppression of normal tissue.

TYPE OF LEUKAEMIAS:
1. Acute
    a. Acute Lymphoblastic.
    b. Acute myeloblastic.
2. Chronic
    a. Chronic Lymphocytic.
    b. Chronic myeloid.

CLINICAL FEATURES:
1. General features like malaise, tiredness, weight loss with lethargy and anorexia are present.
2. Abdominal fullness with pain and discomfort.
3. Breathlessnes on exertion.
4. Spleen is usually palpable and firm in consistency with smooth and painless outline.
5. Hepatomeagly is seen in occasional cases with lymphadenopathy.

Q-8. Define Haemophillia. Suggest 4 Homoeopathic Renedies (1983.)

Ans. HAEMOPHILIA: It is a congenital disorder of coagulation resulting from the deficiency of factors VIII and IX.
1. PHOSPHORUS: It is specially suited to the persons of

thin chest wall with fair complexion and a Tubercular diathesis.

It has a Haemorrhagic diathesis with bleeding under the skin. The blood is usually bright red and coagulable.

2. CROTALUS HORRIDUS: It is good for bleeding diathesis when the blood is dark, non cogulable and offensive. All secretions are blood stained including sweat which is also bloody.
3. MILLEFOLIUM: It is good when bleeding occurs from any and every orifice of the body. It is bright red with soreness of the affected parts.
4. CHINA: See Q-4.

Q-9. Compare and contrast.
a. Hodgkin's and Non Hodgkin's Lymphoma (1991 Supp.)
b. Acute myeloid and chronic myeloid Leukaemia (1991 Supp.)

	HODGKIN'S LYMPHOMA	NON HODGKIN'S LYMPHOMA
1.	It is a painless progressive enlargement of lymphoid tissue with a characteristic histologic finding described by Thomas Hodgkin	It includes the diseases in which uncoordinated growth of lymphoid tissue is present along with normal lymphoid tissues not showing Reed Sternburg cells and without showing destruction of N Lymphoid tissue..
2.	ETIOLOGY: Although uncertain but some infective agent similar to R.N.A virus is responsible.	Here the oncogenic virus is responsible.
3.	Males are predominantly affected.	Both sexes are equally affected
4.	Cervical lymph nodes are first to be affected.	Enlargment of any group may occur
5.	From cervical group of lymph nodes it involves the mediastinum thereby causing the pressure symptoms.	From lymph nodes the spleen, bone narrow and gastrointestinal tract are affected.
6.	PROGNOSIS: is poor.	Is comparitively good.

	ACUTE MYELOID LEUKAEMIA	CHRONIC MYELOID LEUKAEMIA
1.	AGE: Common in children	Common in middle aged and elderly
2.	ONSET: is abrupt	It is insidious.
3.	O/I of Skin: Petechiae + Bleeding Gums + Retinal Haemorrhage	Anaemia + Purpura + Spontaneous Haematemesis
4.	General features: Pallor +++ Tiredness +	Fever + Weight loss + Perspiration increased malaise
5.	Secondary infection like Herpes, Bronchitis, Pneumonia are common.	It is not very common
6.	Organ infilteration occurs early.	It occurs in later stages.
7.	a. Spleen is just palpable b. Liver is much enlarged.	It is massively enlarged Liver may be palpable.

Q-10. Write short notes on

1. **EOSINOPHILIA:** (1977, 1984, 1985, 1987 Supp, 1988.)
   An increase in the total eosinophillic count is called Eosinophillia.

CAUSES:

1. ALLERGIC DISORDERS: Bronchial Asthma, Hay fever, Serum sickness.
2. PARASITIC INFESTATIONS: Hook worm infestations, Ascariasis etc.
3. DRUG ADMINISTRATION: eg streptomycin, liver extracts.
4. SKIN DISEASES: Eczema, Exfoliative dermatitis
5. PULMONARY EOSINOPHILLIA: Tropical eosinophilia, Loeffler's syndrome.
6. BLOOD DYSCRASIAS AND MALIGNANT LYMPHOMAS: Chronic myeloid leukaemia.
7. Following Irradiation.

2. **E.S.R** (1982, 1987, 1988 Supp.)

It measures the sedimentation in mm covered by the upper level of the Red cell column in Ist Hour. It measures the suspension stability of R.B.C and is also a rough measure of abnormal concentration of fibrinogen and S. globulins.

METHODS:
1. Westergrens method
2. Wintrobe's method

The normal value by westergren method in males is 3-10 mm in Ist Hour and in females it is 5-15 mm in Ist Hour.

While the wintrobes method gives the value of 0-9 mm in males and 0-20 mm in females.

E.S.R IS INCREASED: IN:
1. Pregnancy.
2. Anaemias Except Sickle cell anaemia.
3. Acute M.I.
4. R.A.
5. S.L.E.
6. multiple myeloma.
7. Extensive tissue damage.

3. **RH FACTOR.** (1986.) The Rhesus antigen was first discovered by Land Steiner and wiener from the Rhesus monkey.

Persons whose blood gives this reaction have a blood group factor called Rh +ve. If the blood does not give reaction it lacks it and is called Rh-ve.

If a Rh -ve person is transfused with Rh +ve blood the Rh antibody resulting from this may agglutinate the R.B.C of any subsequent Rh +ve blood which may be transfered setting up a Haemolytic reaction.

The Rh grouping should be done before transfusion specially in young females and in mothers who had repeated still births.

4. **LEUCOPENIA:** (1974, 1982, 1986.)

A reduction in the number of leucocytes below the lower limit of 4000/cumm.

CAUSES:

I. INFECTIONS
   a. Bacterial: Typhoid, Paratyphoid, Brucellosis
   b. Viral: Influenza, measles, Infective Hepatitis.
   c. Protozoal malaria, Kala azar.

II. DEFECTIVE BONE MARROW FUNCTION
   a. Aplastic anaemia.
   b. megaloblastic anaemia.

III. BONE MARROW INFILTERATION
   a. Secondary CA.
   b. Malignant Lymphoma.
   c. Multiple Myeloma.

IV. SENSTIVITY TO MANY DRUGS
   a. Chlorom phenicol.
   b. Thio uracil.

V. SHOCK
   a. Traumatic.
   b. Anaphylactic.

5. HYPERSPLENISM: (1991 Supp.)

It can be defined as a Syndrome comprising of Splenomeagly, pancytopenia in the presence of a normal or Hyperactive marrow and reversibility by splenecotmy

TYPES:
1. Primary
2. Secondary to
   a. Congestive splenomeagly.
   b. SABE.
   c. Kala Azar.

CLINICAL FEATURES:
They usually appear as a result of PANCYTOPENIA.
1. Features of anaemia are present.
2. Repeated bacterial infections are seen.
3. Spontaneous Haemorrhages from Thrombocytopenia.

DIAGNOSIS BY
1. By labelling R.B.C and platelets with chromium studies.

TREATMENT: splenectomy.

6. THALASSEMIA (1985)

It is also called Cooley's anaemia. It is found in children

of mediterranean type. It is a rare familial condition in which the osmotic resistance of the R.B.C to Hypotonic saline with fragility are increased.

CLINICAL FEATURES:
1. There are attacks of Haemolytic anaemia
2. Splenomeagly is present.
3. Liver is also palpable.
4. Mongolian Face is due to the bones of the vault of skull being filled with bone marrow.
5. Reticulocytosis is seen.

PROGNOSIS: The full disease leads to death before puberty.

7. **RISKS OF BLOOD TRANSFUSION** (1988.)
   They can be categorised as
   I   DUE TO METHOD OF TRANSFUSION
   1. Acute circulatory failure.
   2. Pulmonary oedema.
   3. Thrombophlebitis.
   II   DUE TO QUALITY OF BLOOD.
   1. Allergic Reactions urticaria, Itching.
   2. Due to old citrate Pyrexial reaction.
   3. Infections due to bacterial contamination.
   III DUE TO ENTRY OF PATHOGENS
   1. malaria
   2. Jaundice
   3. Syphillis

8. **PLATE LET COUNT** (1989.)

They are small corpuscles with basophillic cytoplasm and azo granules in the cytoplasm.

Their normal value is 200,000 - 450,000/cumm.

THROMBOCYTOPENIA: is the count below 150,000/cumm

CAUSES :
1. Idiopathic Thrombocytopenic purpura.
2. Leukaemia.
3. Aplastic Anaemia.
4. Hypersplenism.
5. Drug Reactions.

THROMBOCYTHAEMIA: The count more than 450,000/cumm

CAUSES :
1. Poleythaemia vera
2. After Splenectomy
3. Following acute Haemorrhage.

9. **REED STERNBURG CELL:** (1991)
They are the cells diagnostic of HODGKIN'S DISEASE. They are also seen in
1. Infectious mononucleosis
2. Non Hodgkin's Lymphoma
3. Mycosis Fungoides.

FEATURES: It has abundant eosinophillic cytoplasm and ranges in size from 15-45/UM in diameter.

It is distinguished chiefly by the presence of a multilobed nucleus or with a multinucleus with round prominent Nucleoli

There are 2 mirror image nuclei each containing a large INCLUSION LIKE ACIDOPHILIC NUCLEOLUS which is surrounded by a distinctive clear zone imparting an OWL EYED APPEARANCE.

10. **ACUTE LYMPHATIC LEUKAEMIA** (1987)
This type of leukaemia is more common in children arising from lymphoid tissue.

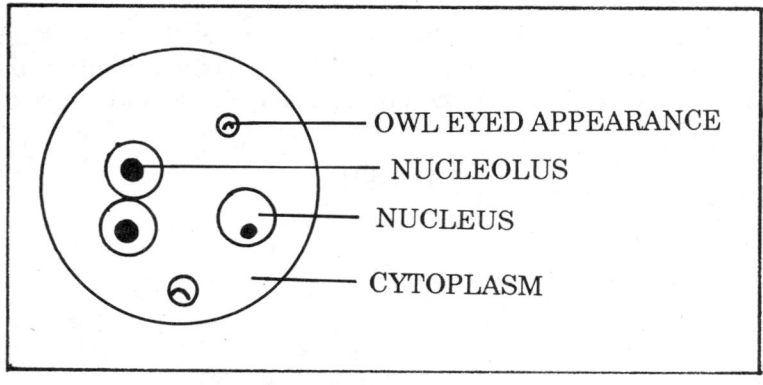

(REED STERNBURG CELL)

CLINICAL FEATURES:
1. Fever, pallor with Lymphadenopathy.
2. Bleeding tendencies are common.
3. Opthalmoscopic Findings show: pallor of optic disc, venous engorgement, haemorrhages and exudates.
4. Neurological Involvement, takes the form of meningitis, cranial nerve palsies, convulsions.
5. Hepatospleno meagly

LAB FINDINGS:
1. Normochromic Normocytic anaemia
2. Platelets are reduced
3. Bone marrow shows infilteration by Lymphoblasts.

11. FACTOR VIII AND IT'S IMPORTANCE: (1992)

It is one of the important components of coogulation system. It is also called Anti Haemophillic factor.

The normal level is 0.5 - 1.50 i.u/ml and is usually measured by a cloting assay.

The propensity to bleeding is related to the plasma factor VIII level, those with levels less than 0.02 - 0.01 I.U/ml as moderate and those with greater than 0.10 I.U/ml as a mild form of disorder.

Its deficiency causes HAEMOPHILLA.

12. CHYLURIA: (1982)

Escape of Chyle through the urine due to rupture of varicose chyle vessels through the mucus membrane of urinary tract is called CHYLURIA.

It gives a milky white colour to urine. It contains fat particles, albumin and fibrinogen Microscopic Examination shows the presence of microfilariae, few R.B.C and lymphocytes.

CAUSES:
1. Filariasis.
2. Rupture of Thoracic duct.
3. Thrombosis in Azygous vein.

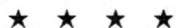

12. CARDIOVASCULAR SYSTEM

Q-1. What are the symptoms and signs of C.C.F.? Mention 4 important drugs in its Treatment. (1988)

Ans. The term congestive failure is applicable to the conditions associated with venous congestion whether systemic or pulmonary. It is a condition characterised by in ability of the Right ventricle to propel the blood forwards resulting in engorgement of (R) atrium, systemic veins with enlargement of liver and dependent oedema.

SYMPTOMS:

I. CARDIAC SYMPTOMS:
1. Palpitation
2. Heaviness of praecordium

II. RESPIRATORY SYMPTOMS:
1. Breathlessness: It usually develops secondary to (L) ventricular failure.
2. Cough with frothy sputum.

III. GASTRO INTESTINAL SYMPTOMS:
1. General Symptoms: anorexia, nausea, vomiting, fratulence, constipation, feeling of tightness over the body with ascites.
2. Hepatic enlargement.

4. URINARY SYMPTOMS:
1. Olguria
2. Nocturia.

5. Swelling of the body: It appears first around the ankle. It is usually noticed after the day's work.

SIGNS

1. Decubitus in propped up position.
2. Resp Rate is increased
3. There is tachycardia

4. J.V.P is raised
5. EXAMINATION OF CVS: Triple Rythm with presence of S_3 and S_4 sounds.
6. EXAMINATION OF ABDOMEN:
   a. Hepatomeagly: Liver is soft and tender
   b. Ascites is present.

HOMOEOPATHIC DRUGS

1. ADONIS VERNALIS: It can be used as a replacement for Digitalis when pulse is slow and weak with cardiac dropsy and scanty urine with anasarca. It prolongs the diastole. There is usually a history of Rheumatic fever with praecordial pain, palpitation and dyspnoea.
2. CONVALLARIA: The heart symptoms are associated with uterine soreness. There is orthopnoea with endocarditis. Feels as if the heart stopped then suddenly started. Valvular heart disease with scanty urine, feeble heart sounds. The patient is worse in a warm room and better in open air.
3. STROPHANTHUS: It is useful in obese persons with weak heart resulting from alcohol, tobacco, coffee or tea.

Heart symptoms with EXOPTHALMIC GOITRE in aged and children. Pulse is quick with breathlessness. Pulmonary oedema and cardiac Asthma with anasarca and scanty urine.

4. ARSENIC ALBUM: It is useful in later stages of heart disease after suppression of measles oedema, restlessness, dyspnoea and suffocation are < after midnight, on lying down.

Irregular Heart, quick beats < in the morning with MARKED PROSTRATION.

Q-2. Describe Cardiomyopathies mention the Homoeopathic medicines used to treat this condition. (1988 Supp.)

Ans. A disease of cardiac muscle of unknown cause and degeneration is called CARDIOMYOPATHY:

CLASSIFICATION:
1. CONGESTIVE CARDIOMYOPATHY:

Cardiovascular System

CAUSES:
1. Systemic H.T 2. Immunological disorders.

Symptoms:
1. Dyspnoea   2. Pain in chest with palpitation

SIGNS:
1. Abrupt jerky arterial pulse of normal volume.
2. Late systolic murmur loudest at the (L) sternal edge and at the apex.
2. HYPERTROPHIC CARDIOMYOPATHY: There is ventricular outlet obstruction with reduced (L) ventricular capacity.

CLINICAL FEATURES:
1. A familial evidence is strongly present.
2. SIGNS ON EXAMINATION:
    a. Jerky, ill sustained pulse.
    b. Late Systolic murmur at the (L) sternal edge and apex radiating into the axilla.
    c. Splitting of P_2 due to delayed closure of aortic valve.
3. RESTRICTIVE CARDIOMYOPATHY. There is obliteration of ventricular cavities with impairment of diastolic filling due to fibrosis of endocardium or in myocardium

CAUSES:
1. Endomyocardial Fibrosis 2. Amyloidosis

CLINICAL FEATURES:
1. (R) SIDED DISEASE: It resembles CONSTRICTIVE PERICARDITIS with increased Jvp, severe ascites and unimpressive ventricular pulsations.
2. (L) VENTRICULAR TYPE OF DISEASE: It produces a mid systolic murmur due to mitral Regurgitation.

HOMOEOPATHIC MEDICINES: See Q-1.

Q-3. Give the causes of Hypertension with it's complications. Mention 4 Homoeopathic medicines. (1988 Supp.)

Ans. When the Blood pressure remains more than 140/90 mm Hg persistently or more as according to the age or sex of the person it is called HYPERTENSION.

CAUSES:
1. PRIMARY OR IDIOPATHIC OR ESSENTIAL H.T.
2. SECONDARY CAUSES:
   a. CARDIOVASCULAR DISEASES: Coarction of aorta
   b. RENAL DISEASES: Glomerulonephritis, Pyelonephritis, Polycystic kidney, Renal artery stenosis.
   c. ENDOCRINE DISEASES - Pheochromocytoma
   - cushing's Syndrome
   - Conn's Syndrome
   - Hyperparathyroidism
   - Acromeagly
   - primary Hypothyroidism
   d. DRUGS: oral contraceptives, Corticosteroids etc.
   e. Alcohol
   f. PREGNANCY: Pre eclamptic Toxaemia.

COMPLICATIONS:
1. HEART DISEASE:
   a. Heart failure
   b. Angina Pectoris.
   c. Aortic dissection
2. MALIGNANT H.T. It is a triad of Papilloedema, proteinuria and Diastolic pressure persistently over 130 mm Hg.
3. Renal DISEASE: Renal damage with proteinuria leading ultimately to Renal failure.
4. Hypertensive Encephalopathy.
5. Cerebrovascular accidents in the form of embolism, thrombosis and Haemorrhage are seen.
6. OCULAR CHANGES: in the form of Hypertensive Retinopathy.
7. HAEMORRHAGES: in the form of epistaxis, Haemoptysis etc.

HOMOEOPATHIC DRUGS:
1. BELLADONA: Headache with redness of eyes, full with throbbing pain < from least jerks but better by pressure, covering the head and sitting errect. Sudden and violent onset of all complaints, with rush of blood to head and face.
2. AMYLNITRATE: It arrest the paroxysms of epilepsy and

Angina pectoris. Olfaction also lowers the B.P. but has a little effect on malignant H.T. Blushing of face with craving for fresh air. There is a sense of constriction with praecordial anxiety.

3. RAUWOLFIA SERPENTINA: There is bursting throbbing headache with giddiness. Haemorrhages like epistaxis, are common with sleeplessness due to Hypertension complaints are usually acute with a sudden onset.

4. AURUM METALLICUM: It is a good Remedy for valvular lesions of arteriosclerotic nature. The pulse pressure is low with palpitations, rapid and irregular pulse. There is ascites with sleeplessness at night. Cardiac pains with Hypertrophy which are worse at night. The patient is depressed, melancholic with self condemnation, worthless feeling, disgust of life and always wants to commit suicide.

All the complaints have a syphilitic backgound.

Q-4. What is left ventricular Failure? Give 2 important causes with management of LVF. (1982, 1988 Supp.)

Ans. LEFT VENTRICULAR FAILURE: It is the failure of (L) ventricle to propel the blood forwards resulting in accumalation of blood in the pulmonary circulation characterised by PAROXYSMAL nocturnal dyspnoea, gallop rythm, pulses alternans and basal creptitations.

CAUSES:
1. Hypertensive Heart Disease (HHD)
2. Valuular Heart Disease (VHD)

MANAGEMENT:
1. Rest in bed in propped up position or back rest inclined at an angle of 45°.
2. USE OF SEDATIVES: to reduce anxiety and decrease the venous retun by causing peripheral vasodilatation.
3. O_2 Inhalation. It is given through the nasal catheter usually but venturimask can also be used.
4. Use of Diuretics: Thiazide derivatives are commonly used.
5. If hypertension is the primary cause then Reserpine 0.5-1 mg I.m is to be injected.

6. If pulmonary oedema is persistent and is resistant to any therapy then Intermittent positive pressure ventillation should be given.
8. Use of vaso dilators like nitroglycerine to decrease the preload or after load.
9. Homoeopathic Drugs : See Q-1.

Q.5. What is C.C.F.? Give the Signs and Symptoms with complications. Write about the management and Homeopathic drugs. (1976, 1977 Supp, 1978 Supp, 1981 Supp, 1987, 1991.)

Ans. COMPLICATIONS:
1. Arrythmia
2. Thrombo Embolism
3. Impaired Liver Functions
4. Hyponatremia
5. Hypokalemia
6. Uraemia

For Signs and Symptoms see Q.1
For management see Q.5.

Q.6. Discuss the Symptoms of Acute Rheumatic Fever. Give It's main Complications. What are the important drugs for it's treatment? (1977 Supp. 1982, 1987.)

Ans. MAJOR CRITERIA   MINOR CRITERIA
1. Carditis   Fever
2. Arthritis   Arthralgia
3. SubcutaneousNodules Previous R.F. or R.H.D
4. Chorea
5. Erythema Marginatum.

COMPLICATIONS:
1. RHEUMATIC HEART DISEASE: In the form of M.S., M.R.
2. Cardiac Arrythmias
3. Pericarditis with effusion.
4. Pneumonia
5. Pulmonary Embolism
6. C.C.F.

HOMOEOPATHIC DRUGS

1. **ACONITE:** There is great anxiety with restlessness fear of death and crowd. Congestion, intolerable and violent onset of complaints.

   The complaints result from exposure to dry and cold winds. There is intense restlessness with increased thirst for cold water.

2. **SPONGIA TOASTA:** It is a good remedy when the cough develops as a reflex of organic heart disease. There is sense of suffocation during sleep which awakes him from it.

   Cough with pain in chest with anxiety and Restlessness. The complaints are usually worse by talking, reading and lying down but better by eating.

3. **KALMIA LATIFOLIA:** The complaints usually results from metastasis of rheumatism to heart. There are severe pains in chest which are associated with numbness and go from above downwards.

   There is palpitation which is worse by leaning forward. There is breathlessness from pressure in epigastrium.

4. **SPIGELIA:** It is a good remedy when complaints result from exposure to cold and suppressed discharges. There are frequent attacks of palpitation with weak and irregular pulse. Breathlessness with inability to lie on (L) side. Must lie on (R) side with Head high.

Q-7. Differentiate mitral stenosis from mitral Regurgitation. Write 3 drugs for each condition with symptoms. (1987 Supp, 1992.)

MITRAL STENOSIS	MITRAL REGURGITATION
1. Narrowing of mitral valve is called in stenosis.	The incompetence of mitral valve is called MR..
2. ETIOLOGY: Rheumatic Fever	- R.F, Endomyo cardial Fibrosis.
3. AGE: Usually seen in young and middle age group.	It can be seen in any age group but particulary in late middle age.
4. SYMPTOMS	
a. Haemoptysis is the prime symptom.	Not seen

MITRAL STENOSIS	MITRAL REGURGITATION
b. Dyspnoea on efforts in later stages with cough.	It is the first symptom to present with; or in the form of P.N.D.
c. Recurrent attacks of Bronchitis.	Not very marked.
5. FACIAL APPEARANCE: Typical mitral Facies with pallor and swelling of face.	Nothing peculiar.
6. PULSE: is usually low volume and regular	It is full, bounding.
7. O/P: a. Apex Beat of Tapping type	No specificity.
8. O/A: a. I^{st} heart sound is loud with mitral opening snap.	I^{st} heart sound is muffled
b. Apical mid Diastolic murmur.	murmur at apical region of PANSYSTOLIC TYPE.
c. No splitting of 2nd sound.	2nd heart sound is split.
d. Third heard sound usually not audible.	It is generally heard.
9. X-Ray, shows predominantly L.A and R.V Hypertrophy with prominent pulminary conus.	Here L.A and L.V Hypertrophy is seen.
10. E.C.G. shows 'P' Pulmonale pattern	It shows 'P' mitral pattern.

SYMPTOMS OF MITRAL STENOSIS:/MITRAL REGURGITATION

1. Exertional Dyspnoea
2. Acute pulmonary oedema
3. Chronic (R) heart failure in the form of ascites, fullness of abdomen etc.

HOMOEOPATHIC MANAGEMENT: See Q-1.

Q-8. Define Angina Pectoris. Write the miasmatic treatment by suggesting 4 Homoeopathic Remedies with

Cardiovascular System

their Indications. **(1984)**

Ans. ANGINA PECTORIS: It is the discomfort resulting from acute myocardial ischaemia.

The word Angina means "I CRY". It is used to denote the cardiac pain of short duration due to inadequate blood supply to the cardiac musculature.

MIASMATIC BACKGROUND: It suggests a PSO-ROSYCOTIC background in operation.

1. CACTUS GRANDIFLORUS: Constriction in chest with a sensation as if the heart were grasped by an iron hand. Cold Sweat and suffocation with gradually increasing and decreassing pains.

   There is constant feeling as if the chest is encaged and each wire is being twisted tighter and tighter. Pains with inability to lie on (L) side. All complaints have a periodicity at 11 A.M.

2. HYDROCYANIC ACID: Feeling of suffocation, pain and tightness in chest. Pulse is weak, irregular with violent palpitations. There are torturing pains in the chest with great sinking sensation at epigastrium.

3. NAJA TRIPUDIANS: Dragging and anxiety in praecordium. Feeling of weight on the praecordium. Patient is depressed with suicidal tendency

   Angina pains radiating to the nape of neck Left shoulder and arm with anxiety and fear of death. Pain in (L) temple is a strong indication.

   Complaints are usually associated with Hypotension, coldness of body, with slow, weak irregular pulse. Pains are associated with OVARIAN NEURALGIA.

4. SPIGELIA: Precordial pains of stabbing shooting lacerating and darting nature. Pains from precordium are reffered to either (L) or both the arms. Dyspnoea with Palpitations which are usually better lying on Right side with head high. Palpitation audible with shaking of chest.

Q-9. Describe the etiology, pathology with clinical features of mitral Stenosis. Write 3 Homoeopathic medicines for it. (1974, 1975 Supp, 1977, 1982, 1983.)

Ans. ETIOLOGY :
1. Rheumatic Fever.
2. SABE
3. Endocardial Fibroelastosis
4. Left Atrial myxoma
5. Congenital: associated with ASD, coarctation of aorta.

PATHOLOGY: In active Rheumatic valvulitis the damage of the valves mostly occurs at the line of opposition; due to trauma during repeated closur. Fibrin and platelets are deposited in that line with fibroelastic proliferation.

The scarring of valves is followed by calcification. The mitral opening may be like a slit as a Button Hole or may further be narrowed down due to shortening of chordee.

For clinical Features and Homoeopathic Drugs.
See Q-7. Q-1.

Q-10. What do you know of myocardial inferction, Angina pectoris? How will you manage such a case. Write 4 Homoeopathic Remedies. (1983.)

Ans. MYOCARDIAL INFARCTION: It is one of the severe forms of IHD.
1. PAIN: Severe pain in praecordium of constricting type which is worse by exertion, by respiratory efforts.
   It radiates to the (L) arm, to the nape of neck, or back between the shoulders.
2. DYSPNOEA: It is variable.
3. NAUSEA AND VOMITING: are common.
4. SHOCK: The patient is cold, pale, or cyanosed. generally profuse sweat with restlessness and anxiety.
5. ASSOCIATED SYMPTOMS: Abdominal destension with epigastric fullness, hiccough, palpitation, dizziness or mental confusion.

ANGINA PECTORIS: The discomfort felt in the praecordium due to acute myocardial ischaemia is called A pectoris.
1. PAIN: is usually felt in the praecordium is severe, of distressing nature.
   Other features of pain are similar to MI.
2. DYSPNOEA: is not usually present.
3. OTHER SYMPTOMS:

a. Choking sensation in throat
b. Belching or passage of flatus
c. Polyuria
d. Dizziness and fainting

MANAGEMENT:
1. Control of Risk Factors: like H.T, Smoking, should be corrected.
2. REST: It is advised these days. But early ambulation is advised to prevent Thromboembolism.
3. RELIEF OF PAIN: Pethidine or morphine should be given subcutaneously.
5. I.V. DRIP: Infusion of 5.% Dextrose is started.
6. If need O_2 inhalations can be given.
7. Phenobarbitone is given to relief the anxiety.

HOMOEOPATHIC REMEDIES: See Q-8.

Q-11. What are the causes of Praecordial pain. Describe the clinical features of a case (1974 Supp, 1978 Supp, 1982.)

Ans. CAUSES OF PAIN:

I   CARDIAC CAUSES :
   1. Angina Pectoris.
   2. MI
   3. Pericarditis

II AORTIC CAUSES
   1. Aortic aneurysm

III PULMONARY CAUSES
   1. Pneumothorax
   2. Pleurisy
   3. Bronchogenic CA

IV OESOPHAGEAL
   1. Reflux Oesophagitis
   2. P.U.S.

V   MUSCULOSKELETAL
   1. Costochondritis.
   2. muscle spasm.
   3. Herpes Zoaster of Inter costal nerves.

VI VASOMOTOR AND ENDOCRINE DISORDERS
   1. ovarian Dysfunctions
   2. Hypertensive Crisis of pheochromocytoma.

VII PSCYHOGENIC: usually seen in nervous, anxious and Hysterical females
For clinical Features: See Q-10.

Q-12. Discuss the clinical features and investigations of Acute pericarditis progressing to CARDIAC TAMPONADE. Write 3 Homoeopathic drugs 1989.

Ans. SYMPTOMS:
1. Pain in chest of dull aching type.
2. Dyspnoea on exertion.
3. Faintness.
4. Pressure symptoms due to effect on surrounding structures like: trachea, lungs, oesophagus.
5. Constitutional Symptoms: like fever, sweating, loss of weight and Fatigue.

SIGNS:
O/I: 1. Patient is seen in the bending forward posture.
2. Localised or a general bulge is seen in precordium.
3. JVP is raised.
O/P: 1. Apex Beat is not felt.
2. Pericardial rub may be felt.
O/Percussion:
1. Upper border of cardiac dullness in 2nd-3rd space when the patient lies flat.
2. Increased cardiac dullness.
3. Impairment of resonance in Cardio hepatic angle.
O/A: 1. Heart sounds are faint and muffled.
2. Pericardial friction rub is present.
3. Bronchial Breathing and aegophony below the (L) angle of scapula.

INVESTIGATIONS:
1. X-Ray shows ular shaped heart shadow with straightening of both (L) and (R) borders.
2. E.G.G.: is low voltage with inverted T waves.
3/ Angocardiography: reveals a gap usually of about 3-5 mm caused by the thickened pericardium.

HOMOEOPATHIC DRUGS:
1. CACTUS: See Q-8.

Cardiovascular System

2. KALMIA: See Q-6
3. SPIGELIA: See Q-6

Q-13. Describe the management of a case of acute C.C.F following M.I. (1991 Supp.)

Ans. There are 3 aspects of the management of Cardiac failure.
1. Eradication of the precipitating and the fundamental cause.
2. Improvement of cardiac output and efficiency
3. Treatment of consequences

IMMEDIATE MANAGEMENT:
1. Relief of pain by morphine or pethidine.
2. Rest.
3. use of sedatives to reduce anxiety.
4. Intensive coronary care admission.
5. Administration of O_2 Inhalations.
6. Use of Diuretics.
7. Use of Digitalis therapy.
    For Further details Refer to Q-4.

Q-14. Discuss the causes of Aortic Stenosis. How will you investigate and manage such a case. Give 4 Homoeopathic Renedies. (1992.)

Ans. The narrowing of aortic value due to causes of varying etiology is called AORTIC STENOSIS.

ETILOGY:
1. Rheumatic
2. Congenital
3. Calcified Bicuspid valve
4. SABE
5. Hyperlipidaemia
6. Senile.

INVESTIGATIONS:
1. Chest X-Ray:
2. E.C.G: Shows features of LVH with LBBB or A.V Block.
3. Cardiac Catheterisation: Shows a pressure gradient of

more than 60 mm of Hg across the aortic valve
4. Echocardiography: To assess the (L) ventricular function.

TREATMENT:
1. Medical management has no role.
2. Prophylactic pencillin, diuretics and salt restricted diet are helpful before surgery.
3. INDICATIONS OF SURGERY:
    a. Recurrent attacks of Syncope
    b. Progressive (L) vent failure.
    c. Recurrent original pain not due to coronary disease.

HOMOEOPATHIC DRUGS:
1. NAJA : See Q-8.
2. HYDROCYANIC ACID : Refer Q-8.
3. CONVALLARIA MAJUS : See Q-1.
4. ADONIS VERNALIS : See Q-1.

Q-15. Discuss the Risk Factors of coronary Artery Disease. What is Angina Pectoris. Describe it's medicinal Treatment (1992.)

Ans. RISK FACTORS:
1. HYPERTENSION: It carries the increased risk of IHD
2. Cigarette Smoking.
3. Obesity
4. Hyperchloesteraemia: With increased serum lipids.
5. Heredity: It is common in people with blood group A and there is a definite Familial relation.
6. AGE AND SEX: There is preponderance of males; now no age is exempt from it.
7. DIABETES MELLITUS:
8. OTHER RARE FACTORS
    a. Early menopause in women.
    b. Hyperuricaemia
    c. Physical Inactivity
    d. Polycythaemia.

For 2nd part See Q-8.

Cardiovascular System

Q-16. What are the leading symptoms of cardio vascular diseases? Give with examples. (1983.)

Ans. 1. DYSPNOEA: It can be either dyspnoea on exertion or on lying down called ORTHOPNOEA.
It can be graded into the following.
1. GRADE I: Able to do Housework or job with difficulty.
2. GRADE II a. Comfined to chair or bed but able to get up with moderate difficulty.
   b. Confined to the chair or bed and only able to get up with great difficulty.
3. GRADE III: Totally confined to the bed or chair.
4. GRADE IV: Even at Rest.
2. PAIN IN CHEST
3. PALPITATION: Can be felt as chirping of birds in chest. It is usually worse by motion.
4. SYNCOPE: Frequent fainting attacks. It can be associated with dizziness, sweating, pallor, pain, diarrhoea, fever and Haemorrhage.
5. GIDDINESS: usually seen after mental or physical exertion.
6. GASTRO INTESTINAL SYMPTOMS MANIFESTED IN A CVS CASE: Nausea, vomiting, Diarrhoea, Abdominal fullness.
7. URINARY SYMPTOMS: oliguria with difficulty in passing urine.
8. LOSS OF WEIGHT: Especially in children.

Q-17. What is Heart Block? Describe its varieties and give the Clinical picture of complete Heart Block with its treatment. (1976, 1977 Supp.)

Ans. The delay or interruption of the conduction of Impulses from the SA node along the (N) pathway to the ventricular myocardium results in Heart Block.

TYPES:
1. SINOATRIAL BLOCK: The impulses arising from the SA node are blocked at the junction of SA node with the atrial musculature and hence the beat is missed.
2. ATRIOVENTRICULAR BLOCK: It is caused by the abnormalities at the A.V Junction or along the His purk-

inje system. It may be seen in the following forms:
a. Ist Degree Heart Block: Clinically it is asymptomatic except E.C.G shows lengthening of PR Interval
b. 2nd Degree Heart Block.
c. 3rd degree or complete Heart Block: In this the impulses fromthe SA node are totally interrupted from reaching the ventricular muscle.

SYMPTOMS:
1. The patient complaints of frequent attacks of syncope on least exertion but sometimes even at Rest.
2. Palpitation on exertion.
3. Dimness of vision with a sinking feeling.

EXAMINATION:
1. Pulse, is slow and low volume.
   No other evidence is seen clinically.

TREATMENT:
1. Although the prognosis is poor but still the PACE MAKERS are inserted. If good quality lead can be connected to it, the chances are far better.
2. Homoeopathic Drugs like Digitalis, Kalmia and Apocyanum can be tried.

Q-18. Write Short Notes on
1. **AORTIC STENOSIS** (1987)
   See Q-14.
2. **HYPOTENSION** (1987 SUPP.)
   When the systolic B.P remains below 90-100 mmHg it is called Hypotension.

ETIOLOGY:
1. A Hereditary condition
2. Cardiac Diseases like LVH and failure, Coronary Thrombosis.
3. Addison's Disease
4. Pulmonary T.B
5. Cachexia
6. Exhausation mental or physical
7. Shock, Collapse, Haemorrhage

SYMPTOMS:

It usually presents with vague symptomatology like
1. Headache
2. Giddiness
3. Syncope when rising from recumbent posture
4. Depression
5. Lassitude
6. Undue Fatigue.

In case of POSTURAL HYPOTENSION the Systolic B.P is 20-30 mm less when the patient is standing than when lying down.

TREATMENT:
1. Diet should be good and nourishing.
2. Free purgation, Very hot baths and prolonged standing should be avoided.
3. Undue mental and physical strain should be avoided.
4. Use of vasoconstrictor drugs.

3. **ANGINA PECTORIS:** (1987 Supp)
See Q-8, 10.

4. **ARTERIOSCLEROSIS** 1987 SUPP, 1991

It is a degenerative disease of the arteries of which the different types as mentioned below are recognised.
    a. Atherosclerosis
    b. Medial Sclerosis including moncke berg's type.
    c. Arteriolar Sclerosis.
    d. Hypertension.

It usually starts as a patchy thickening of the intima of large arteries. It is often found in early adult life but becomes more marked after the middle age.

It is closely related to lipid metabolism. It can occur at a very early age in Diabetes, in Nephrosis, myxoedema and obese patients.

SIGNS:
1. Thickened and palpable arteries.
2. Increased pulse pressure with a rise in Systolic B.P.
3. An alteration in 2nd Aortic sound.
4. Irregularity of the calibre of Retinal vessels with obstruction to the outflow.

5. **APOPLEXY:** (1987 Supp.)
   See Q-18 of Nervous system.
6. **CARDIAC OEDEMA:** (1983.)
   It is mainly due to diminished cardiac output giving rise to a fall in filteration pressur in the Renal glomeruli. It results in the retention of sodium ions by osmosis of water.
   It starts in the most dependent parts as in the lower part of the back when lying or in the ankle when ambulatory.
   In the H/O the case dyspnoea will have preceeded the Complaint.
   Oedema with Heart failure is called CCF. Oedema in the absence of dyspnoea is not due to cardiac disease.
7. **APEX BEAT** 1976, 1982, 1983.
   The most distinct and outermost cardiac impulse felt in the 5th intercostal space just inner to the midclavicular line is called APEX BEAT. It is a palpatory finding of CVS examination.

TYPES OF APEX BEAT:
1. TAPPING: It is seen in RVH. Where on palpation the beat strikes and goes away.
2. HEAVING: It is seen in LVH which is characterised by a SUSTAINED IMPRESSION OF BEAT ON PALPATION.

CAUSES OF DEVIATED APEX BEAT: To (L):
1. Pleural Effusion or Pneumothorax on (R) side.
2. Fibrosis or callopse on the (L) side
3. Hypertrophy or dilatation of Heart

DEVIATED TO (R)
1. Pleural effusion or Pneumothora on (L) side.
2. Fibrosis or collapse on (R) side
3. In A.S.D rarely

IMALPALPABLE APEX BEAT
1. Thick chest wall
2. Emphysema
3. Pericardial Effusion
4. Overlying the rib
5. Obesity with pendulous breasts.

8. **WATER HAMMER PULSE:** (1977 Supp, 1980, 1983, 1983 Supp)

Cardiovascular System

It is a large bounding pulse assoicated with increased stroke volume of the (L) ventricle and decrease in peripheral Resistance leading to a wide P. Pressure.

The pulse strikes the palpating finger with a rapid foreful jerk and then quickly disappears.

It is best felt in Radial artery with the patients arm elevated.

CAUSE OF THIS: It is caused by the sudden emptying or artery.

CAUSES:

I PHYSIOLOGICAL
  1. Fever
  2. Alcohol
  3. Pregnancy

II PATHOLOGICAL
  1. A.R
  2. P D A
  3. Systolic H.T
  4. Thyrotoxicosis
  5. Cirrhosis of liver
  6. Cor pulmonale

9. **BRADYCARDIA:** (1982.)

When the countable heart rate is below 60/min it is called BRADYCARDIA.

ETIOLOGY

1. In athletes
2. Myxoedema
3. Digitalis Therapy
4. Raised Intracranial pressure
5. Sinus BradyCardia
6. Third degree or complete Heart Block.

10. **P WAVE** 1989.

It is produced by atrial depolarisation. It is best visualised in Lead II and normally does not exceed 3 mm in height or 3 mm Horizontally. It is upright in all leads except aVR.

ABNORMALITIES:

1. ABSENT: In Atrial fibrillation, SA block.

2. INVERTED IN LEAD I: Dextrocardia.
3. WIDE AND NOTCHED: P mitrale in (L)ATRIAL enlargement.
4. TALL AND PEAKED: P pulmonale in (R) Atrial enlargement.

11. **OPENING SNAP** (1991.)

It is the diagnostic of M.S. It is heard best at the apex shortly after the 2nd sound. It usually indicates the degree of Stenosis.

Shorter the interval between 2nd sound and opening snap tighter is the Stenosis.

CAUSE:

It is caused by the sudden flapping back of the mitral cusps when th rapidly falling Left ventricular pressure falls below the Left atrial pressure.

The opening snap is absent if the valve is rigid or calcified.

12. **Differentiate Benign from malignant H.T** (1991 Supp)

BENIGN H.T	MALIGNANT H.T
1. ONSET and presentation is insidious, for years long duration.	It has a dramatic presentation.
2. AGE: It usually occurs in persons above 50 yrs.	can be seen in any age but more in young age.
3. RANGE OF B.P: Diastolic above 100 mm Hg	It is above 130 mm of Hg.
4. Family History is usually +ve.	No definite Family History
5. PATHOLOGY: There is increased arteriolar resistance of unknown mechanism.	Diffuse arterioler sclerosis with partial obliteraby fibrinoid degeneration
6. CLINICAL FEATURES	
a. Asymptomatic ·	Papilloedema is the Ist presentation.
b. Vague symptoms like suboccipital Headaches, fullness, lethargy, lassitude	It may present as Haematuria or Renal

BENIGN H.T	MALIGNANT H.T
with giddiness.	failure.
7. PROGNOSIS when diagnosis is established it is comparitively good.	Poor prognosis.
8. RESPONSE TO ANTIHYPER-TENSIVES: is good.	Not seen.

13. **HEART BLOCK:** (1974 Supp)
See Q-17.

14. **VENTRICULAR TACHYCARDIA** (1992.)
It is one of the forms of PAROXYSMAL Tachycardia. It is seen usually in old age.

ETIOLOGY:
is usually unknown.

SYMPTOMS:
1. Onset is sudden with severe palpitation.
2. Fluttering sensation in the Heart.
3. Dizziness or Syncope.
4. Praecordial pain with Breathlessness.

SIGNS:
1. The Heart and pulse rate varies from 150-250/min and is regular.
2. It is a fixed pulse as it is not infuenced by change of posture or exercise.
3. Carotid sinus massage may terminate the tachycardia.
4. E.C.G : QRS wide complexes with bizzare pattern and P waves are not clearly seen.

15. **RHEUMATIC CARDITIS** (1992.)
It is a pancarditis involving the pericardium, myocardium and the endocardium. It is seen in about 40-50/- cases of R.F. It is one of the earliest manifestations of Rheunatic fever.

SYMPTOMS: Pain in Praecordium with dyspnoea.

SIGNS:
1. Presence of friction rub indicative of pericarditis.
2. Presence of mitral or mitral and Aortic regurgitation

3. Features of myocarditis:
    a. Cardiac Enlargement
    b. Soft Ist Sound
    c. Carey Coomb's murmur.
4. Features of Endocarditis:
    a. Presence of pansystolic murmur of MR.

16. **ATRIAL SEPTAL DEFECT** (1992.)

The patent foramen ovale is the ASD. It is more common in females.

PATHOLOGY: Since the (N) Right ventricle is much more compliant thanthe (L) a large amount of blood shunts through the defect fromthe (L) to (R) Atriumand hence to the (R) ventricle and pulmonary arteries.

CLINICAL FEATURES:
1. It is asymptomatic untill the pul obstruction occurs then it manifests in the form of dyspnoea, cardiac failure and arrythmia.
2. **SIGNS.**
    a. Wide Fixed Splitting of 2nd Heart Sound.
    b. A Systolic murmur over the pulmonary area.
    c. Loud P$_2$ in pulmonary area.
    d. Systolic Thrill

COMPLICATIONS:
1. Pulmonary Hypertension.
2. RVH.
3. Reversal of shunt.

★ ★ ★ ★

13. INFECTIOUS, TROPICAL AND DEFICIENCY DISEASES

Q-1. Discuss the clinical features and Signs of Diptheria along with Differential Diagnosis. Mention important drugs used in the treatment. (1977, 1978, 1980, 1982, 1983, 1987, 1988 Supp)

Ans. The following are the important clinical features:
1. ONSET: is usually sudden
2. CONSTITUTIONAL SYMPTOMS: Malaise, fever, debility, lethargy are very well marked.
3. ANTERIOR NASAL DIPTHERIA: There is either unilateral or bilateral discharge which is often blood stained, later becomes thick, mucopurulent and foul smelling. Redness, excoriation, small follicular spots or pustules are present on the upper lip.
4. FAUCIAL DIPTHERIA: There is excessive salivation with low grade fever, cough and irritation of throat.
5. PHARYNGEAL DIPTHERIA: There is marked irritation of throat with congestion and cervical lymphadenopathy.
6. LARYNGEAL DIPTHERIA: There is brassy cough with hoarseness of voice, noisy breathing and progressively increasing laryngeal obstruction.

SIGNS OF DIPTHERIA:
1. The fauces are congested with a band of redness around the Tonsillar edge. There is a thick greyish white membrane which is present with small multiple spots, when removed it bleeds easily.

DIFFERENTIAL DIAGNOSIS:
1. Follicular Tonsillitis.
2. Infectious mononucleosis.
3. Quinsy.

4. Acute Bronchiolitis
5. Foreign Body in Larynx.

HOMOEOPATHIC MEDICINES:

1. LAC CAN: It is good for Diptheria with the formation of membrane on (L) side with pains on affected side which constantly shifts from one place to another. Shining glazed appearance of deposit with pearly white membrane. Throat feels burnt, raw better by cold drinks.
2. BELLADONA: Throat is dry as if glazed with angry looking congestion; red, worse on (R) side. Throat feels constricted with difficult deglutition, worse by liquids. Continous inclination to swallow with a scraping sensation.
3. LACHESIS: The complaints are on (L) side with dusky bluish appearance of membrane. Pain in throat aggravated by Hot drinks. The throat is very painful and worse from slighest pressure, touch is even more annoying.

Q-2. Discuss the main features of patient with Kalaazar. How would you diagnose? Give 4 drugs (1985, 1987)

Ans. Kala azar is a common tropical disease caused by the protozoal parasite Leishmania Donovani.

1. ONSET: Can be either enteric or malarial or it can be insidious with ill health and lassitude
2. GENERAL APPEARANCE: The patient is emaciated with dry and sparse Hairs, pigmentation around malar bones and temples, around the mouth with protuberant abdomen, thin legs and oedema of feet.
3. ALIMENTARY SYSTEM:
    a. Spleen: is non tender and palpable.
    b. Liver is painless and is felt on palpation.
    c. There is usually good appetite with chronic Diarhoea.
    d. Jaundice can occur ocasionally.
4. FEVER: There is double diurnal rise of temperature lasting for 2-6 wks followed by a phase of Apyrexia.
5. GENERALISED LYMPHADENOPATHY: The lymph nodes are soft and non tender.

Infectous, Tropical and Deficiency Diseases   235

6. HAEMORRHAGES: are usually noticed.

HOMOEOPATHIC REMEDIES:

1. CROTALUS HORRIDUS: It is good for Kala azar when haemorrhages are usually associated. The liver and spleen both are enlarged. The urine is dark with casts. All the lymph nodes are enlarged. Patient is aggravated by lying on (R) side and in open air.
2. CHIONANTHUS: It is a good remedy for splenic fevers with aching in umbilical region with a feeling as if a string is suddenly drawn.

Clay colored stools with palpable liver with PERIODICAL ATTACKS OF HEADACHE.

3. CEANOTHUS: It is good for Kala azar with markedly enlarged and palpable liver and spleen. There is pain in (L) side with violent dyspnoea. Unable to lie on (L) side.
4. MYRICA: There is dull pain in the region of liver and spleen with loss of appetite but with a constant feeling of fullness in abdomen.

The patient is very despondent, irritable and gloomy.

Q-3. Describe malaria. Give its varieties and causative organism. Suggest 4 Homoeopathic drugs required (1986.)

Ans. It is a common tropical Disease caused by the species of Plasmodium variety.

INCUBATION PERIOD: 10-15 days.

CLINICAL FEATURES:

1. ONSET: is sudden with lassitude, headache, chilliness several days before the actual attack.
2. PAROXYSMS: It can be divided into 3 clinical stages.
    a. COLD STAGE: There is shivering with chills and rigors, Chattering of teeth and he covers himself with blankets. It lasts for about half hour and temperature goes on rising.
    b. HEAT STAGE: Shivering reduces and gives place to a feeling of intense heat with a desire to throw away all the coverings. Face is flushed with dry and burning skin, headache and vomiting.

It lasts for about 3-4 hours.

C. SWEAT STAGE: During this stage he breaks into profuse perspiration which gives a feeling of relief with lowering of temperature.

TYPES OF MALARIA:
1. VIVAX MALARIA: The characteristic intermittent periodic fever becomes established only in the later stages
2. QUARTAN MALARIA: The intermittent periodic fever starts from the begining.
3. FALICIPARUM MALARIA: It usually does not show all the 3 paroxysms of chill, heat and sweat.

HOMOEOPATHIC MEDICINES:
1. CHININUM ARS: There is intense periodicity of complaints with weariness and prostration. Head feels full with throbbing and anxiety. There is alternation of hyperacidity and decrease of acid and anorexia.

    Intense chilliness with weak limbs, coldness of hands and feet is very marked.
2. ALSTONIA: It is generally indicated in late stages i.e. the stage of sweat with great exhausation Malarial fever with diarrhoea, dysentry and feeble digestion. It is also used as a tonic after exhausting fevers.
3. CINCHONA: It is a good remedy for complaints resulting from exhausting discharges and loss of vital fluid with nervous erethism.

    Fever Paroxysms return every week with all the 3 stages well represented.

    Patient is chilly in the afternoon, it commences in breast with thirst before chill.

    There are debilitating night sweats with free perspiration on every little exertion especially on single parts.

Q-4. What is Scurvy? Describe its causes and manifestations. Outline the general management with 3 Homoeopathic medicines. (1982, 1985.)

Ans. SCURVY: It is a deficiency disease resulting from the deficient intake of vitamin C.
1. ONSET: is usually gradual with fretfulness, increasing pallor or tenderness of legs.

Infectous, Tropical and Deficiency Diseases

2. DUE TO HAEMORRHAGES:
   a. Under the periosteum of Long Bones. There is usually PITHED FROG POSTURE with thighs flexed and abducted and Knees flexed.
   Infilterations of muscles with blood leading to oedomatous limbs.
   b. GUMS: They usually bleed easily from least trauma.
   c. Petechiae on the skin
   d. Within the orbit there is bleeding leading to PROPTOSIS.
   e. Haematuria usually microscopic.
   f. Blood in stools.
3. Anaemia
4. Low grade fever is common.

MANAGEMENT:

1. Intake of Vitamin C: Fresh fruits and vegetables in the quantity of 3-4 ounces.
   Ascorbic acid 100 mg is required

HOMOEOPATHIC MANAGEMENT:

1. MERC SOL: There is foetid odour from mouth with increased salivation. The gums are spongy, bleed easily with receding margins.
   Sore pain on touch and from chewing. Tongue is flabby with imprints of teeth.
2. KREOSOTE: It is equally efficient in the cases of scurvy specially with painful dentition. The gums are bleedy and Spongy with rapid decay of teeth. They crumble easily.
3. ACETIC ACID: It is also good for scurvy with a bleeding diathesis and the blood is generally bright red. It causes soreness with great prostration after Haemorrhages.
   There is profuse salivation with dribbling of saliva throughout the day.

Q-5. What is the etiology, clinical features and types of Dengue fever? Give 3 Homoeopathic drugs. (1985)

Ans. It is a tropical disease of viral etiology **CAUSATIVE**

AGENT: Group B arbo virus is responsible. It is transmitted by the female mosquito Aedes Aegypti.

CLINICAL FEATURES:
1. STAGE OF INVASION: Sudden onset with malaise, severe headache, pain in eyeballs, intense pain in joints and muscles with bodyaches; which is aggravated by movements.
Face is flushed with congested eyes, photophobia and ocasionally nausea and vomiting.
2. STAGE OF REMISSION: On about 3rd day temperature drops to normal and remains so, for about 12 hrs to 3 days. Patient feels well in general.
3. STAGE OF TERMINAL FEVER AND ERUPTION: During this period recurrence of pain and fever with appearance of rash all over the bdoy except face is seen.
4. STAGE OF CONVALESCENCE: Fever subsides by 6th or 7th day, pains diminish and gradually disappear. Joint pains and other sequale may persist for a short period.

CLINICAL TYPES:
1. Typical Break Bone type.
2. Enteric Type.
3. Encephalitic Type.
1. EUPATORIUM PERFOLIATUM: It is a good remedy when bone pains are very marked with PERIODICITY at about 7 A.M. Chill with body aches and soreness preceeded by great thirst. Nausea, vomiting at the close of chill with throbbing headache.
Perspiration relieves all the complaints except headache.
2. GELSEMIUM: It is good when the complaints result from being overheated or in sun for a long time. The chill is very violent and it shakes the person. Chills go up and down along the back with great muscular soreness and prostration. Heat and sweat stages are exhausting. Complete thirstlessness with dullness, dizziness and drowsiness.
3. BRYONIA: There is aching soreness in each and every muscle. The pains are aggravated from least motion but

better by pressure and by complete rest. There is increased thirst for large quantities at longer intervals. Complete dryness of mucus membranes is remarkably seen.

Q-6. Name 3 diseases where Hyperpyrexia is found. Give the clinical features and management of any one of them. (1982 Supp.)

Ans. HYPERPYREXIA: 1. malaria.
2. Pneumonia
3. Influenza.
MANAGEMENT OF MALARIA: See Q-3.

Q-7. Describe the clinical features of whooping cough. What are its complications? Name 4 Remedies. (1976, 1983, 1984.)

Ans. It is one of the infectious diseases caused by the microorganism Bordtella Pertusis.

CLINICAL FEATURES:
They can be divided into 3 stages.
1. CATARRHAL STAGE: Insidious inonset with coryza moderate or mild cough and slight fever. The cough is at first in single paroxysm then becomes very intense.
2. PAROXYSMAL STAGE: The paroxysms usually follow with repeated episodes of short staccato cough. During the paroxysm face is red or deeply cyanosed with bulging tearful eyes.

There is vomiting of food debris after paroxysm of cough.
3. CONVALESCENT STAGE: About the 4th week the paroxysm is diminished in intensity with general improvement.

COMPLICATIONS:
I RESPIRATORY COMPLICATIONS:
   1. Pulmonary atelectasis.
   2. Bronchopneumonia
   3. Hilar adenitis
   4. Asphyxia.

II. CENTRAL NERVOUS SYSTEM
   1. Convulsions.
III. PRESSURE EFFECTS:
   1. Rise in Intraabdominal pressure with development of Herniae and prolapse of Rectum.
   2. Rise of Intrathoracic pressure with subconjunctival haemorrhage.
   3. Pneumothorax.

HOMOEOPATHIC REMEDIES:
1. Drosera Rotundifolia.
2. Merc cynatus.
3. Pertussin.
4. Hyoscyamus Niger.

Q-8. Describe the causes and manifestations of Filariasis. Mention the complications with Indications of 4 Remedies.   (1984.)

Ans. Filariasis is a tropical disease caused by wucheria Bancrofti.

CLINICAL FEATURES:
1. FILARIAL FEVER: usually high fever with rigors, nausea and vomiting are common.
2. INFLAMMATORY PHASE:
   a. Acute Lymphangitis. of the lower extremities with fever rigors and toxaemia.
   The tender, inflamed lymphatics are seen as red streaks. It is accompanied by itchy, irregular erythematous swelling of the skin.
   b. Lymphadenitis: The glands are swollen, firm and tender commonly in the groins and supratrochlear area.
3. LATE OBSTRUCTIVE PHASE: following inflammatory reactions is common.
   a. Lymphatic varices. are prominent in the region of femoral, inguinal and testicular areas.
   b. Chyluria
   c. Elephantiasis with thickening of overlying skin.

Infectous, Tropical and Deficiency Diseases

COMPLICATIONS:
1. Chyluria.
2. Recurrent Infection.
3. Abscess formation in any part due to dissemination of emboli.

HOMOEOPATHIC DRUGS:
1. HYDROCOTYLE: Skin is dry with thickening of epidermoid layer. Intolerable itching specially of soles. Elephantiasis of syphilitic origin.
2. ELAEIS: Elephantiasis associated with thickened skin, itching and complete anaesthesia of the skin.
3. ARSENIC ALBUM: It is good when there are burning pains in the limbs with great swelling and enlarged, painful lymph nodes.

Pains are associated with restlessness and anxiety. There is increased distress from pains which are usually worse at Night.

Q-9. Name the preventable diseases of Childhood. Discuss in detail the Immunization schedule. (1990 Supp.)

Ans. There are certain diseases prevalent in childhood which if prevented can save the child from the risks which are generally operable.

They are:
1. measles.
2. Diphtheria.
3. Whoping cough.
4. Tetanus.
5. mumps.
6. T.B.
7. Poliomyelitis.
8. Typhoid (although questionable)..

BENEFICARIES	AGE	VACCINE	NO OF DOSES	ROUTE OF ADMINISTRATION
Infants	6 wks to to 9 months	DPT	3	I.M
		Polio	3	oral
		B.C.G	1	intradermal

BENEFICARIES	AGE	VACCINE	NO OF DOSES	ROUTE OF ADMINISTRATION
	9-12 months	measles		Subcutaneous
Children	16-24 months	D.P.T	1"	I.M
		Polio	1**	Oral
	5-6 yrs	DT	1@	I.M
		Typhoid	2	Subcutaneous
	10 yrs	T.T	1@	I.M
		Typhoid	1@	Subcutaneous
	16 yrs	T.T.	1@	Subcutaneous
		Typhoid	1@	Subcutaneous
**:-		BOOSTER DOSE		
@-2Doses		If not	Vaccinated	properly

Q-10. Discuss various types of Leprosy with it's treatment. (1988 Supp.)

Ans. Leprosy is an infectious disease caused by the mycobacterium Leprae. It can be of the following types

1. **TUBERCULOID LEPROSY:**
   a. Nerve Lesions: The patient complaints of sensory and or motor symptoms depending on the type of nerve involved. Usually a single and superficial nerve is affected like greater auricular, ulnar nerve, median nerve etc.
   b. Skin Lesions: Early presentation is the presence of macules usually few and asymmetrically distributed over the body particularly over the arms, legs and buttocks.

   They have well defined edges with Hypopigmented borders. There is complete loss of sensation, of touch over them. Anhidrosis or abscence of sweat is a peculiar feature.

2. **LEPROMATOUS LEPROSY:** It usually commences with the appearance of macules on the skin. They are symmetrically distributed having an ill defined edge. The symptoms can be seen under:
   a. Nasal: Nasal blockage, discharge and bleeding from the nose.
   b. Eyes: Attacks of Hazy vision with pain and redness of eyes. They show punctate Keratitis.
   c. Face: It is called LEONOINE FACIES where there is thinning of eyebrows, broad or deformed nose,

Infectous, Tropical and Deficiency Diseases

thick ear lobes, falling of upper central or lateral incisor with Hoarseness of voice.

There is glove and stocking anaesthesia with shortening of fingers due to repeated trauma.

3. **BORDERLINE LEPROSY:** It can be
   a. Borderline Lepromatous: Nerve involvement occurs early as compared to the skin lesions.
   b. Borderline Tuberculoid: Lesions are few with hair loss and absence of sweating.

TREATMENT:

1. Chemotherapy: Triple drug therapy of Dapsone, Rifampicin and clofazimine is advocated.
2. Rest and sedatives.
3. Surgical Treatment.
   a. Excision of small lesions.
   b. Removal of necrosed bone with splitting of nerve sheath.
4. Homoeopathic drugs like Hydrocotyle, Aurum met, Arsenic album, Hoang nun etc can be used.

Q-11. Describe Protein calorie malnutrition. Give its management. (1988 Supp)

Ans. PROTEIN CALORIE MALNUTRITION: is a syndrome due to deficiency of proteins, calories or both.

ETIOLOGY:

1. Insufficient feeding.
2. Infections and infestations.
3. Bad social customs and prejudices, poverty and poor personal habits.

MARASMUS:

It develops from the absolute or relative deficiency of both calories and proteins

1. The weight of the child is less.
2. Development is retarded.
3. Severe loss of subcutaneous fat from all over the body.
4. Limbs are cold and body temperature is subnormal
5. Monkey like face is commonly seen
6. Muscles are flabby with Hypotonia.

7. Child constantly cries with intercurrent infections.
8. The milestones are usually delayed with features of underlying disease may be present.

KWASHIORKOR:
It results from the deficiency of proteins.
1. It is usually seen in breast fed infants where the deficiency appears after the weaning is started.
2. Skin is shining due to oedema; with erythematous and pigmented patches.
3. Hairs are day, brittle and lustureless.
4. Liver is generally enlarged, non tender and soft.

TREATMENT:
1. GOOD DIET: Diet rich in proteins, calories, vitamins and minerals is necessary. Milk or milk substitutes are given.
2. DEWORMING: It is essential to control the underlying infection.
3. TREATMENT of underlying causes.

Q-12. Discuss in brief the symptoms of infestation with roundworms. What preventive measures can you suggest to prevent the disease from occuring in the community? What are its complications. Mention with names only 4 drugs. (1987 Supp.)

Ans. **CLINICAL FEATURES:**
1. MECHANICAL EFFECT: Due to mechanical irritation there may be abdominal pain, nausea, vomiting, loose motion, abdominal distension. Rarely mechanical obstruction of the gut, appendix may occur.
2. TOXIC EFFECT: This effect is due to an allergen called Ascaron released by Ascarias. It gives rise to urticaria, fever, Bronchitis, ascariasis pneumonia.
3. NUTRITIONAL EFFECT: Features of malabsorption of fat, Carbohydrates anaemia, puffiness of face are seen.
4. NEUROLOGICAL EFFECT: Cerebral irration with grinding of teeth and Convulsive seizures.

PREVENTIVE MEASURES:
1. Avoidence of raw vegetables or fruits. If want to take

Infectous, Tropical and Deficiency Diseases

then they should be washed in Potassium permangnate solution.
2. Use of metronidazole as a prophylactic atleast 2 times a year.

COMPLICATIONS:
1. Obstruction of intestines, billiary tract and Respiratory tract.
2. Pneumonia
3. Perforation of Typhoid ulcer
4. Appendicitis.
5. Peritonitis.
6. Intususception.

HOMOEOPATHIC DRUGS:
1. Cina
2. Santonine
3. Spigelia
4. Teucrium.

Q-13. Write short notes on
1. **SCURVY** (1988)
   See Q-4.

2. **PELLAGRA** (1988, 1989, 1991 Supp.)
   It is due to deficiency of nicotinic acid characterised by diarrhoea, dementia and dermatitis.

CLINICAL FEATURES:
1. SKIN: Erythema symmetrically appear on exposed parts of body especially on the back of hands wrist, forearm. There is redness, swelling and itching.
   There may be cracking, exudation and ulceration in acute cases. Skin changes around the neck is called CASTLE COLLAR OR NECK COLLAR.
2. G.I.T: Tongue is raw, beefy red, painful and swollen with hypertrophic papillae of tongue. Angular stomatitis with cheliosis are common Nausea, burning sensation in epigastrium with diarrhoea.
3. NERVOUS SYSTEM: In mild cases there is anxiety weakness; depression, mental dullness, apathy and irritability. In chronic cases there may be amnesia with

degeneration of posterior and lateral columns of spinal cord.

TREATMENT:
1. Diet should be rich in proteins.
2. Nicotinic acid should be taken orally
3. Diarrhoea should be adequately controlled.

3. **THREAD WORM INFESTATIONS:** (1988.)

These worms are called OXYURIS VERMICULARIS.
MODE OF INFECTION: Infection occurs due to ingestion of eggs which contain larvae. These larvae escape into upper intestines and become matured.

CLINICAL FEATURES:
1. Diarrhoea, itching of the perianal skin, urethral irritation, vaginal discharge and nocturia.

TREATMENT:
Homoeopathic Drugs like Chelone, Sanotnine, Ratanhia can be used. ːrazine salt is given for 2 weeks.
2. Personal cleanliness is very important.

4. **ROUNDWORM INFESTATIONS:** (1983, 1988 Supp)
See Q-12.

5. **SCABIES:** (1988 Supp)
See Q-6 under skin.

6. **KOPLIK'S SPOTS:** (1982 Supp.)

They are a diagnostic feature of measles. These tiny whitish or bluish white spots appear in the mucus membrane of mouth on the 2nd day of infection. They appear as TINY TABLE SALT CRYSTALS against a reddish background.

They are seen maximally near the opening of parotid duct at the level of upper 2nd molar teeth. They may also appear on the medial conjunctival folds and also on the vaginal mucous membrane.

They disappear before the appearance of true rash.

7. **COMPLICATIONS OF MEASLES:** (1991 Supp.)
The following are the complications.

I **EARLY COMPLICATIONS:**
1. Secondary bacterial otitis media.
2. Pneumonia or Bronchopneumonia.
3. Laryngotracheobronchitis or croup.

Infectous, Tropical and Deficiency Diseases

    4. Encephalitis.

II **LATE COMPLICATIONS**
    1. Bronchiectasis.
    2. Immunosuppresive encephalopathy
    3. Subacute Sclerosing pan encephalitis.

8. **HEAT STROKE** (1988 SUPP.)

Heat Hyperpyrexia or sunstroke is also named as Heat stroke. It is characterised by sudden loss of consciousness which may be preceded by prodromal signs of cerebral Irritaion like headache, dizziness, nausea, convulsions and visual disturbances.

Failure of heat regulating centre gives rise to high fever and cessation of sweating.

ON EXAMINATION:
1. Skin is hot and flushed with dryness.
2. Pulse is rapid, irregular weak with low B.P.
3. Temperature is between 105-107°F.
4. Ultimately the features of hyperpyrexia may be seen.

MANAGEMENT:
1. Cooling by fanning after sprinkling with water
2. Immersion in cold water or use of ice packs.
3. massage of extremities to maintain circulation.
4. Normal Saline 1000 ml I.V slowly if dehydration or cramps appear.

9. **COMPARE CHICKEN POX WITH SMALL POX (1991 SUPP, 1992.)**

CHICKEN POX	SMALL POX
1. It is a disease caused by varicella group of virus i.e. by Herpes zoaster virus.	It is caused by virus resembling that of vaccinia andcowpox antigenically.
2. Age/Sex: It chiefly affects the children under 10 yrs of age.	It may affect anyone without any predilection for sex.
3. Incubation period is from 14-21 days.	It is from 7-21 days
4. Constitutional features are mild and short lasting.	They are severe and long lasting.

CHICKEN POX	SMALL POX
5. Distribution of rash is Centripetal.	It is centrifugal more on the limbs and periphery than on the trunk.
6. Differt types of lesions appear at the same time.	The lessions usually follow each other within a coarse of time.
7. Eradication: It has not been eradicated	It has been eradicated under WHO's small pox eradication programme.
8. Complications are rare.	They are severe
9. The lesions are vesicular without leaving any marks.	They are pustular and leave behind the pox marks.

10. Compare marasmus and Kwashiorkor (1991 Supp.)

KWASHIORKOR	MARASMUS
1. It is an infantile disease seen commonly due to proteins deficiency.	It is due to both proteins and calorie deficiency.
2. General Appearance oedema with moon shaped face.	Progressive loss of weight with sunkeness of face and eyes the typical MONKEY FACE.
3. Mental changes like apathy retardation with late in learning to sit and walk in late stage.	They usually appear early in the disease.
4. G.I.T: Diarrhoea with offensive watery stools is common.	constipation is a significant feature.
5. SKIN: oedema with erythema which soon changes into patchy pigmentation is common.	No oedema But skin is loose, dry, lustureless with depressed fontanelles.
6. Hairs are discoloured and brittle in early stages.	They usually appear early
7. TREATMENT: use of proteins, early weaning with mixed diet.	Adequate intake of calories, proteins, fats and minerals with correction of anaemia and intercurrent infections.

11. **BITOT SPOTS** (1984.)

They are a diagnostic hall mark of Vlt A deficiency affecting the eyes. These spots are first seen in the bulbar conjunctivae which gives a smoky appearance. They are triangular in shape and adherent to underlying conjunctivae.

12. **RUBELLA** (1988 SUPP)

It is an infectious disease caused by the Rubella group of virus. It is usually spread by droplet infection and is more severe in adults than in children.

INCUBATION PERIOD: 2-3 weeks.

SYMPTOMS:
1. Fever: rarely exceeds 38°C and does not persist beyond 48 hours.
2. Headache with body aches all over the body.
3. Anorexia, nausea and vomiting with arthralgia.

SIGNS:
1. Temperature is raised
2. Bradycardia
3. Face is flushed.
4. Rashes appear on the Ist or 2nd day of the disease and take the form of small pink macules or papules.
5. Generalised Lymph adenopathy is present.

The whole illness ends in 2-3 days. There is no staining or desquamation of skin.

13. **RICKETS:** The metabolic disorder resulting from the deficiency of vitamin D is called Rickets.

SYMPTOMS:
1. Restlessness more during sleep
2. Irritability
3. Sweating in the forehead specially during sleep
4. Flabby falty child.

SKELETAL DEFORMITY:
1. Enlargement of Costochondral junction with the apppearance of Ricket Rosary.
2. The head is large with prominent frontal and parietal

bosces like HOT CROSS BUN.
3. Dentition is delayed with protuberant abdomen.
4. SPINAL DEFORMITIES: like hyposis, Kyphoscoliosis, knock knee develop.

TREATMENT:
1. REQUIREMENT: is 1200-2000 I.U/day
2. It should be given in the form of cod liver oil, of vitD. Shark liver oil, fortified milk.
3. Exposure to sunlight.
4. Calcium supplements should be given.
5. Massive doses of vitamin D in the dosage of 600,000 I.U should be given by I.M route.
6. Homoeopathic Drugs: like calc carb, calc Flour, sillicea, can be used.

14. **NIGHT BLINDNESS:** (1987 Supp 1991.)
Night blindness or Nyctalopia means defective vision in dim light. It is due to deficiency of Vlt A. It can also be seen in congenital absence of rods, Retinitis pignientosa, Syphilitic retinitis, hysteria, fatigue and anxiety.

15. **HOOK WORM AND IT'S TREATMENT** (1985, 1986, 1988 Supp.)
Hook worm disease in man is produced by Ancylostoma duodenale and Nectar americans.

CLINICAL FEATURES:
1. DURING MIGRATION:
   a. Creeping eruption is produced when the larvae wander about through the skin in aimless manner. It is called GROUNDS ITCH.
   b. Cough, dyspnoea, rusty sputum due to Bronchitis and Bronchopneumonia.
2. ON REACHING THE G.I.T.
   a. Gastric upsets in the form of nausea, vomiting, diarrhoea and gastric distension.
   b. Geophagy
3. Anaemia.

TREATMENT:
1. Correction of anaemia.

Infectous, Tropical and Deficiency Diseases

2. Use of specific drugs like Thymol, Chenopodium and Carbon Tetra chloride can be used.

16. **BLACK WATER FEVER** (1982 SUPP)

It is a condition of rapid intravascular haemolysis associated with chronic Plasmodium Falciparum infection specially when the attacks are recurrent, irregularly treated and suppressed by quinine.

SYMPTOMS:

1. Fever comes with rigors at the onset.
2. Aches and pains in body specially in loins and abdomen.
3. Patient passes urine having a PORT WINE COLOUR.
4. Restlessness. pallor, coldness of extremities are common.
5. In severe cases uraemia develop with anuria and Hiccough.

SIGNS:

1. Temperature is usually high
2. Anaemia and jaundice due to haemolysis
3. Spleen is palpable and tender.
4. There is oliguria and of port wine colour.

TREATMENT:

1. Complete Rest.
2. High Carbohydrates are given.
3. Use of Cortico stersids to arrest Haemolysis.

17. **AIDS** (1992.)

It is a serious and fatal disease characterised by widespread damage to the immune system of the body with susceptibility to unsual cancers and severe infection caused by a virus called HTLV III LAV OR ARU.

SPREAD BY:

1. Close sexual contacts
2. Parenteral transmission through blood and plasma products.

INCUBATION PERIOD: It varies from 6 months to 6 years may be more.

CLINICAL FEATURES:

1. The disease starts slowly with low grade fever and evening sweats.
2. marked weakness and tiredness lasting for several weeks.
3. Anorexia, nausea, vomiting, diarrhoea with weight loss are common.
4. Headache with blurring of vision, delirium may be seen.
5. Respiratoy complaints like cough, dyspnoea, pain chest may develop.

DIAGNOSIS BY

1. Demonstration of virus from blood and different body fluids
2. Low lymphocyte count with low I helper cell count.
3. Screening test from presence of antibody against the virus by ELISA test and WESTERN BLOT KIT TEST. There is no cure at present.

18. **MICROILARIAE** (1989.)

The embroys of wucheria Bancroffi are called microfilariae. These embryos find their way into the blood through the lymph nodes.

SIZE: They measure about 290 mm in length by 6-7 mm to breadth. When dead and stained with Romanosky's stains it shows the following.

1. HYALINE SHEATH: It is a structureless sac which is best seen where it projects slightly beyond the extremities. It remains as an investing membrane round the larva.
2. CUTICULAR CELLS: It lines the sheath in the form of cuticle.
3. SOMATIC CELLS OF NUCLEI: They appear as granules in the central axis of the body and extend from the head to the tail end. At the anterior end there is a space devoid of granules called cephalic space.
4. GENITAL CELLS: A few genitals cells are seen posteriorly in front of thepore.

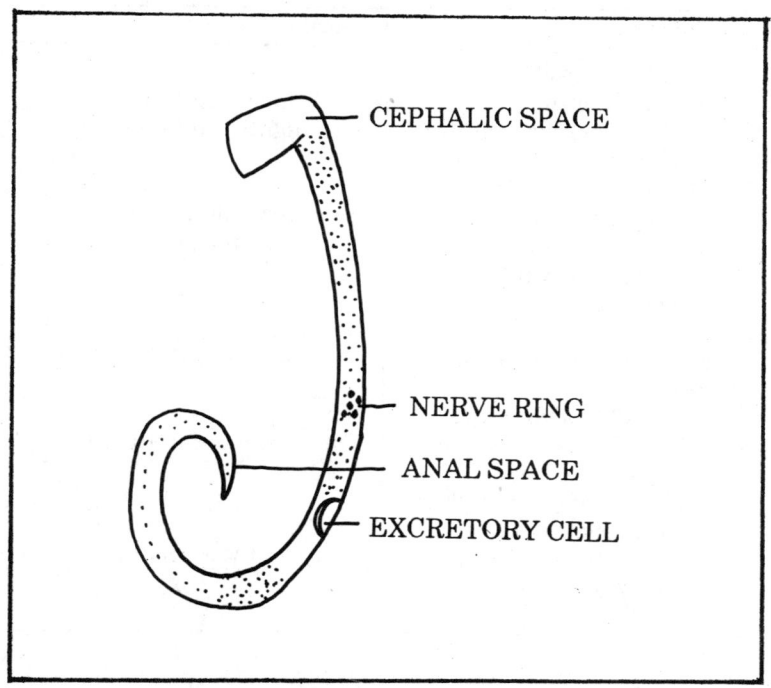

(MICROFILARIA)

19. COMPARE VIRAL AND TYPHOID FEVER (1992)

	TYPHOID	VIRAL FEVER
1.	ETIOLOGY: It is caused by gram +ve salmonella Typhii	It is caused by a group of viruses specially Para Influenza group.
2.	INCUBATION PERIOD: 10-14 days.	1-2 days.
3.	COARSE OF DISEASE: Lasts for atleast 4-6 weeks.	It is usually self limiting within 7-8 days.
4.	PRODROMAL ILLNESS: is less marked in the form of malaise, bodyaches.	It is very marked in the form of violent body aches, sneezing and upper Resp infection.

TYPHOID	VIRAL FEVER
5. MODE OF INFECTION: Orofaecal Route	By droplet infection.
6. PULSE: There is Relative bradycardia.	It is slightly on higher side.
7. PATTERN OF FEVER: It is a step ladder pattern with increase in evening and comes down by morning	It usually follows a pattern of Intermittent fever
8. CONSCIOUSNESS: is affected in the form of delirium	Not seen
9. DEBILITY: is very marked.	Not very well seen
10. RELAPSES: are less with adequate treatment.	They are more frequent.
11. VACCINATION: usually it is given at the age of 6-9 months and at the age of 10/16 yrs.	No role of Vaccination.

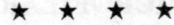